SURVIVING

NORMAL

By

Sonja Brewer

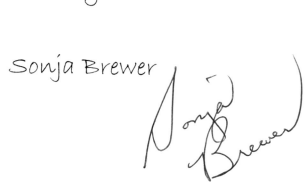

Aventine Press

Published by Aventine Press
750 State St. #319
San Diego CA, 92101

Library of Congress Control Number: 2009931268
Library of Congress Cataloging-in-Publication Data

ISBN: 1-59330-595-8
Printed in the United States of America.

For
Lisa and Kristin

In Memory of
Peter, David, Bob, Bernie, Noreen

Acknowledgments

I thank David's doctors, nurses and caregivers, the hospital staff at Cape Cod Hospital, Whidden Memorial Hospital, the Bedford VA Hospital, Eagle Pond Rehabilitation and Living Center, Comfort Keepers, Alzheimer's Services of Cape Cod and the Islands, Elder Services of Cape Cod and the Islands, the Orleans Council on Aging Day Center and the Brewster Council on Aging transportation service. I particularly thank the staff of the Chelsea Soldiers' Home, a Massachusetts veterans' facility, where skilled nursing and nurturing are a combined standard of excellence that should make all veterans proud. I thank the amazing ministers who helped shine the light of God on otherwise difficult days and some amazingly intuitive social workers who, as a group, offered me a level of empathy that truly kept me going through trying times.

I am also grateful to those who stood tall when it came to offering courage, support, mentoring and love. I thank my daughters, Lisa and Kristin, most of all for their steadfast faith in me and for their exemplary courage in facing such an extended and difficult personal loss. I thank Jack, David's caregiver, for his devotion and for his continuing friendship. I thank the Smith family for lending me Bernie's fierce loyalty and support. I thank the members of our Early Onset Support Group at Alzheimer's Services. I gathered enormous strength and resolve not only from our meetings, but also from our shared dinners and camaraderie. I had forgotten how to care by the time I attended my first meeting, but they restored me and gave me strength.

I thank Connie for her wonderful editing skills as well as her instant recognition that this has been a living project subject to divine control.

I thank the many people who continue to devote their professional lives to research and to, hopefully, finding a cure for this disease.

Fight on.

Foreword

Disease is just a normal part of aging, right? We get wrinkles and gray hair. It gets a little harder to see, a little harder to hear. We don't seem to have as much energy as we used to have. When we start to get a little forgetful, it's not surprising. It's expected, anticipated even. After all, there are many mid-life adults out there tending to their aging parents and this is all just part of the norm.

✦ ✦ ✦ ✦ ✦ ✦

You run into someone you know at the grocery store and in response to the proverbial exchange of "How's it going?" you may reply:

"Oh, fine. Except I'm getting so tired trying to keep up. You know my father has Alzheimer's Disease? Yeah. I've been going over to his house every day to make meals and clean up, only he doesn't want any help. He certainly doesn't seem to want *my* help. But he doesn't have a choice anymore, so neither do I. I can't just leave him on his own. I don't know. Being a caregiver in addition to everything else, I just don't have any time anymore."

"Oh, I'm so sorry to hear that. I can imagine how difficult it must be." (There's that instant understanding.)

"Yes, it's really hard."

"And how old is he?"

"Eighty-two."

"Ah, well... You know, my father had Alzheimer's Disease too. He was eighty-four. We had to put him in a nursing home because it just got too much to take care of him."

"We're starting to look at nursing homes now."

"Well, good luck. I'll be thinking of you."

"Thanks."

And so we move on, back to our busy lives with our holiday planning, vacations, children, friends, shopping, jobs, worrying about paying for college tuitions, planning for retirement. We'll mow our lawns, pay our mortgages and mark the calendar for a visit to Grandpa in the nursing home. He may not appreciate our visit. Hard for the kids. But still, there is that sense of responsibility.

So many families affected by Alzheimer's Disease. We all understand it so well. We know the words. We know what they mean. We instantly know all the frustrations lying just behind those words when someone in our family, usually an aging parent, is diagnosed with this disease.

But then there is this variation of Alzheimer's Disease called *Early Onset Alzheimer's Disease* or EOAD. This aberration of the disease that hits younger people—people under 65. People in their 50s. Even people in their 40s! EOAD is a scary old person's disease that descends smack into the middle of those busy lives with holiday planning, vacations, children, friends, shopping, jobs. It's been more recently referred to as Younger Onset Alzheimer's Disease.

Now, when you meet up with a friend at the supermarket and do the exchange of "How's it going?" it sounds a little different.

"Well, things have been difficult for us. My husband has Alzheimer's Disease."

"Your husband? Oh, you're kidding. I never would have guessed. Why, I just saw him at the library a few days ago. He was laughing and joking. He had some books in his hands. He seemed fine. We had a nice conversation."

"Yes, well… Good, I'm glad to hear that. Yeah, I know. You mostly wouldn't know it. Good. Yeah. Ah. Gotta run. Talk to you later." And the other person continues on, thinking what a shame it is that your 52-year-old husband is sometimes forgetful. Don't we all have our *senior moments*? After all, how could he have driven himself to the library if he had Alzheimer's Disease for real? How could he have joked around and talked coherently? How could he read a book if he really had Alzheimer's Disease? *Nope, that wouldn't be possible. What on earth is this woman talking about?*

This form of Alzheimer's Disease looks normal on the outside. Why not? There is no choice but to go on with your busy life for as long as possible, because that is your life. You are not retired. You are not spending your time playing bingo at the senior center. You are not living a sedentary life at home watching TV.

9

You are doing the things that everyday younger families do, trying to hold on for as long as possible to that normal life. You are still working, shopping, and yes, even going to the library.

In reality, the disease is crushing you and your family, extinguishing every part of what has so far defined you. The person you meet at the store should have conjured up a different image. Would this help?

"Did you know that my husband is ill? Yup, well, it's like cancer, only not cancer. It's kind of a mental illness and a physical illness all rolled into one. He is paranoid, delusional, sometimes psychotic. He has a multiple personality disorder. Sure, you see a nice guy at the library. He can turn on a dime and become mean, aggressive, nasty. Did you know that he couldn't figure out how to put his shirt on this morning? Do you know that he'll probably be wearing diapers in a few years and he will no longer be able to speak or walk?

"Now do you get it? My husband has a terminal illness and we are falling apart. It may not look that way to you because he is still driving around. In reality, we are a mess. We are living day to day with something none of us understands or is equipped to deal with. The fact that he looks normal, so healthy and handsome, well, don't let that make you think he is not sick. He is sick. We are all sick. How can you just go on shopping?"

So that is what I really want to say or maybe scream to get the other person's attention, to get her understanding. But of course, I don't. I move on quickly to relieve the person of the task of ever understanding what such an illness means at such a young age. It's not the time or the place.

✦ ✦ ✦ ✦ ✦ ✦

Well, this is the time and this is the place. This is a story of our lives over the seven-year period that we all suffered with the Early Onset Alzheimer's Disease diagnosis that targeted my husband at an early age. We did the best we could in a world that thought that we were mostly living normal lives. We did the best we could in a world that has boxed an understanding of Alzheimer's Disease into an increasingly normal part of aging.

It is not normal at any age, and it is truly scary when it strikes a relatively young person in the prime of life. Alzheimer's Disease is a terminal illness that can be a threat to younger people. It leaves medical and social services in the dust, bewildered, unequipped to respond in truly helpful ways. It straps families with unimaginable financial and emotional hardships with no relief. It begs for better understanding, better resources and more research. For whatever contribution our story may provide toward those goals, I am thankful, and David would be thankful too.

Sonja Brewer

What lies behind us and what lies before us are tiny matters compared to what lies within us.

— Ralph Waldo Emerson

Year One

I am the unwitting partner in a marriage that is disintegrating, in a relationship that is painful, and in a lifetime that has no more beginnings. You can't choose to be just an observer. No, this is an illness that demands full-blown participation. "In sickness and in health" no longer applies to us because there is really nothing healthy left of us. The "we" of us is gone because we are now joined in sickness, not in health. This is a very contagious illness. It sickens both partners and compromises the best of intentions and the holiest of vows. We await an agonizingly slow and untimely death to eventually "do us part." Sadly, this is what our marriage has become.

Did I really buy into this when I got married so many years ago? I think not. How can anyone know what the future will bring? How we would change over the years. How illness would change us, sometimes in insidious ways. No, I could not have known then what I was committing myself to, and I certainly could not have predicted what strengths might or might not carry me through. That's the reality of it. No one really knows what he or she is capable of until adversity hits.

While I have such great sympathy and empathy for other couples living with illness and disability, being caught in the web of Early Onset Alzheimer's Disease seems particularly cruel. David may rarely admit to his limitations, but deep down he knows and he's angry. Rightfully so. I'm ready for a second lifetime of new adventures, but that's not going to happen. I'm angry too. My adventures will be juggling my job with my role at home as caregiver. I already feel unequal to either task. I totally admit to feeling burdened and depressed over this whole thing. But it is what it is. I'm not going anywhere, so I have to figure this out.

Together we seem to have built a tag team of alternating love and support with mutual anger and resistance. We have our good days and we have our bad days.

This is not a journal. It is a journey. Come with me if you want to. I will dip back a bit to catch you up to date, and then we will move forward together. I know what I've heard. That it's a terrible disease. But what about us? We are young and strong. Maybe it will be different for us.

From what I know so far, I can guarantee that you will find out things that just don't fit into a normal life and just don't fit anyone's explanation for what one could or should expect in a situation like this. I also know that from the outside looking in, we look like any other mid-life couple enjoying and living our lives. This will be a journey, however, from the inside looking out.

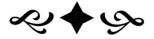

It's late January. We have had a light snow overnight and I see that it powders and drifts over the doorstep as I let the dogs out. Little paw prints dot the back yard as the dogs and I make our way to the fence. I have left David behind in our warm and cozy bed. He rarely gets up with me anymore. Most mornings now, he sleeps. Sometimes he will actually push me out of the bed. I have to go to work and he's glad. He's glad to be rid of me for the day.

I walk the dogs around the boat that looms large over us on its wooden blocks. How long do blocks last before they sink into the earth beneath? For two years now the boat has caught snow and rain, but no waves. It lies dormant waiting for David to rebuild the cabin or replace the engine. In reality, it lies dormant waiting for David to get out of his bad mood.

Over the winter, he spends his days doing nothing. Well, not really nothing. He has his routines and his lists. This is the difficult period, when David is on layoff from his job as an assistant harbormaster. Lucky that we live on Cape Cod. So lucky for a Texas boy who loves the ocean. The job is a wonderful match for his gregarious nature as he maneuvers his work boat from yacht to yacht, smiling and exchanging greetings with his seasonal public each day. It's also a great match for his technical skills and education after 20 years in the Navy and Coast Guard.

The only drawback is the five months of winter layoff that leave him marooned, empty and silent in the house, mostly alone.

It used to be a wonderful reprieve for him. Now, although he regards it as his right to do what he wants, I worry.

The lists are growing in number. They are on the counter, the kitchen table, the bookcase and in the bedroom on the nightstand. Some are old, some new, many rewritten a number of times. The number of lists is starting to get confusing. It's what we need at the store—"bread, ketchup, dog cans, soda, cookies." It's the ingredients for a dinner recipe—"mushroom soup, onions, chicken, paprika." It's what needs to be done—"fix the shower, clean the shed, find the snow shovels." The notes are carefully and neatly written in fine black felt-tip marker on paper from yellow ruled pads. If David cannot find the right pen or the right paper, he will spend the morning looking for it before writing on anything else or before writing a note at all.

I find it strange that David has developed routines that have an element of rigidity and an air of self-importance. Over the past few years, it seems that his winter world has grown smaller and smaller. After sleeping late, he spends most of the day in the kitchen now, hour after hour, sitting at the table or working at tasks that he can do right there in the kitchen. He drinks coffee—lots of it—so along with all the other dishes, the coffeepot has to be carefully washed out and coffee remade at least once or twice during the day. Some days he will use a special coffeepot cleaner to really clean the pot and rinse it out several times.

Dishes are done in a ritualistic fashion using gloves with extremely hot water. We live in a very old house and we don't have a dishwasher. David washes everything in the kitchen sink including cat and dog cans, plastic containers and cleaning brushes. He washes the kitchen floor once a day or once every other day.

Like the dishes, the daily crossword is a careful ritual with the dictionary, Scrabble game, word charts and a pad of paper spread around to assist him. He prints a certain way, always using pen. Never fills in just a few letters of a word. Never crosses anything out. While he has always been quite good at this, completing most crosswords that he starts, it seems that more recently he is only getting halfway through before carefully folding the crossword page and setting it on a shelf to work on later. A stack of unfinished crosswords now sits on the shelf next to his books, boat magazines and lists. They cover the cabinet and chair right beside the table where David sits along with at least 50 pens and pencils gathered from all over the house.

The laundry area takes up the back wall of our large country kitchen. The TV remains on all day, and tuned in to FOX or CNN. David listens while he puts clothes in the washer or sorts and folds clothes on the kitchen table. He lets the dogs in and out from the back kitchen door. It's usually late in the day when he finally leaves the house for a while to walk the dogs or go to the store.

The purchasing is becoming a problem. Why does he seem to be buying the same thing every day? I look in the refrigerator and there are two packages of hamburger meat with a third defrosting. I look in the cupboard and there are four bottles of ketchup. He often overbuys and then he does not follow it up with any care to ensure that we can eventually eat what he buys. If he buys four meats, they all sit on the refrigerator shelf together and the next night, he will go out to buy something else. If I ask for something, he buys two or four. It's never just one.

I should be glad that he goes to the store, I guess. To me it's a chore and I don't look forward to it at all, so I should be happy that David does this. Why do I think he does nothing when he in fact does a lot? It's that what he does is small and petty and all done in a confined space. I find that weird. I find him lazy. The shed does not get cleaned. The shower still drips in the bathroom. The snow shovels are still buried out back somewhere. When I arrive home from a nine-hour work day, there is no dinner waiting for me. David has spent the day in the kitchen and he is still there, staring into the TV. The dogs have not been fed. He wonders why I'm angry.

It seems to me that we are veering off into different directions and most of the time, I don't know what to think. I don't know if David is becoming obsessive-compulsive or, more likely, depressed and in need of medication, or am I being petty? It's the middle of winter. What else should he be doing if he's not working?

Of course, I had no idea at this time that there was a disease that was working hard behind the scenes to destroy his brain-cell connections. I had no idea that he was already struggling and that other brain cell synapses were probably working overtime, sapping his energy, as they tried mightily to keep up. It would be another five months before he would be diagnosed.

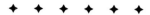

It's February and David seems to have one obsession—himself. Maybe I have been subconsciously aware of the changes in him for quite some time. I knew that we were drifting apart in a hundred different ways, but maybe that's what happens when you have been married for over 30 years. Maybe you just get tired of each other. One person metamorphoses into something the other person cannot relate to and so the choice is to either fight against it or let it happen. I let it happen, thinking it was the normal course of things. I had my interests. David had his. If he wanted to spend his days sitting around, then fine. I would just continue on until he came to his senses.

From the start though, this particular winter layoff period seemed different. It seemed unhealthy from the start and it only got worse. This was more than the two of us drifting apart. This was my husband and life partner descending into some kind of abyss that was so foreign to me that the only thing I knew how to do was to criticize him and complain constantly, thinking my attitude would somehow wear him down and snap him out of it. I am ever so slowly emerging from my own winter solstice now and suddenly becoming an observant and caring person.

✦ ✦ ✦ ✦ ✦ ✦

While I was busy living with and absorbing David's depression, it was not so apparent to me that his memory problems were, in fact, becoming serious problems. I felt immune, as though it really did not affect me. He was someone who wasn't into doing much of anything, who was focused only on himself and, of course, focused on these piddly little things in the kitchen.

For someone like that, adding in a loss of short-term memory rang no alarm bells in me. Why would he care to remember anything for himself or anyone else? It seemed to fit right into the big picture of his changing personality. That changing personality spoke volumes to me that he just didn't care about other people anymore. And of course, it seemed to specifically revolve around me. He did not care about me anymore. Or so I thought.

"Someone called for you." David tells me as I squeeze through the door from work, arms full of papers, shopping bags and my purse.

"Oh, who called?" I ask.

"They didn't tell me their name."

"Well, who didn't tell you their name? Was it a man or a woman?"

"I think it was a woman."

"You can't remember if it was a man or a woman?"

"A woman. It was a woman."

"So where's the message?" I ask, my frustration showing. "Where's the message you're supposed to write down when someone calls?"

"I'm not your personal secretary. Why don't you stay home and take your own calls?"

"Ahh, well, someone has to work around here," I reply, knowingly slinging on the ammunition.

"Right. Like I don't work. I work all day long while you sit around at a desk all day."

"I don't sit around all day as you characterize it. I was out the door at seven a.m. while you were still in bed and I've worked hard all day long. It's common courtesy to take a message."

I want to scream. Again, to me this is a lack of concern and caring for me, a coldness that has settled in over David that is not only frustrating but hurtful, and, in my mind, purposefully so. We have an ongoing pattern of David taking phone calls and simply forgetting to tell me about them, or writing half a scribbled note that I might find on the top of his dresser several days later with an unintelligible name or number.

Now David is ready to go to the store to pick up something for dinner, but he can't find his keys. This is getting to be a habit. I help him look for them. Eventually, I find them in the pocket of a jacket he had put on yesterday when it was warmer. Today, it's cold. Early February. Why do I have to do his thinking for him when I have been thinking hard all day and he has been thinking of nothing at all?

✦ ✦ ✦ ✦ ✦ ✦

Lisa, our older daughter, comes to the Cape for a visit in March. She teaches at a charter school in Cambridge and lives in Boston. Her relationship with her dad is always light, friendly and fun. She has infinite patience, but she remarks to me about Dad forgetting to say that she had called to say what time she would be down.

"Dad, you didn't tell Mom that I wouldn't be here for dinner," she says, smiling at her dad.

"What? Yes, I did. I told her."

"No, you didn't tell me Lisa called," I say.

"Oh, I didn't? I'm sorry. I thought I did."

"It's okay, Dad. No big deal."

Lisa is always so understanding. I am boiling with frustration most of the time, but David could forget a hundred things before Lisa would appear frustrated. Still, she is curious. *Why is Dad always forgetting things?*

Kristin, our younger daughter, is a nurse. We see her more often because she lives nearby, and so she is becoming gradually more aware of the changes in David.

"What's with all these lists, Mom?" Kristin picks up some of the notes David has left on the counter.

"Oh, you know, Dad's lists. He has nothing else to do, so he writes lists," I reply.

"That's not it, Mom. You know that's not it. Dad forgot that he agreed to watch Devon on Thursday. Didn't he leave you stranded at the car dealership last week? He loses his keys all the time. He's forgetting everything. Mom, he has to go to the doctor."

"Yeah, I know, and it's not that I haven't talked to him about it. He should go, but there's no way I'm going to make him go. He hasn't seen a doctor in ten years!"

"No, Mom. What if he has a brain tumor? What if something is really wrong?" Kristin persisted. "He has to go. If he won't call to make an appointment, then I will."

"Well, you can try, but I bet he won't go even if you do make him an appointment."

Kris was true to her word. Before the week was out, David had an appointment with a primary-care doctor listed on his insurance card who had actually never seen him before. He was just a name on a card. David didn't necessarily have a disrespect for doctors, he just felt he had no need for a doctor, so why go. Good for Kris. Coming from her, it was apparently not something that David could ignore. Or maybe it was just because she arranged it, not me. After all, I am David's antagonist. Since Kris arranged it, he agreed to go. I was amazed.

✦   ✦   ✦   ✦   ✦   ✦

So, on a cold day in late winter, David finally saw this doctor he had never seen before. When he was asked why he had made the appointment, he very quietly told the doctor that he was having trouble remembering things. My jaw dropped at how easy it was for him to tell the doctor, yet he had never discussed it in any meaningful way with me. In fact, he had mostly ignored all of our comments about his forgetfulness, frequently joking about it. He would blame us for losing his things sometimes in a laughing and joking manner so that we would all laugh about it. Sometimes, though, it seemed that he really did think that one of us had walked off with a favorite pen or favorite pad of paper, or favorite CD, and you could see his frustration and anger.

So here it was, after all this time, in one sentence quietly delivered to a doctor he did not know. It became real in those very few seconds. It became even more real when this young doctor took him seriously, did a full physical with blood tests, ordered an MRI and neuropsych testing, and gave him a referral to a neurologist.

And as I think about it now, why wouldn't he? Sitting before him was an athletically trim, good-looking, very tanned and healthy-looking young man, a man who looked much younger than his 52 years. His brown hair had only a slight sprinkle of gray on each side, barely noticeable. Yet this was a man with memory problems, perhaps also suffering from depression. The doctor asked me a few questions and I realized that I was not ready to answer them. I mentioned a few things that troubled me about David like his forgetfulness, lack of focus, lack of caring and inactivity. The doctor said that I would be asked more questions by the neuropsychologist so I might want to think about it some more. He must have felt my reluctance. I would now have to give this some attention, since all of a sudden it had the fleeting blessing of reality. And add to that,

David didn't seem to be fighting me. He sat right there with the doctor and listened to what I had to say.

Had my apathy been part of the problem? Why hadn't I pushed David much harder to see a doctor?

✦ ✦ ✦ ✦ ✦ ✦

Over the next few days, I did think about it some more. What should I remember to relate to the neuropsychologist when we meet?

Well, I should remember to say that depression runs in David's family. His brother and sister were both on anti-depressant medication at times, and his brother had committed suicide only five years earlier. This had been extremely hard for David, of course. He was the one who had called from Massachusetts to send the police to his brother's apartment in Texas to check on him when we did not hear from him for a few days. David knew that he had been feeling low. Suicide is unbelievably damaging to family members. It left David angry and sad. It would make sense that he would still be depressed over this.

I should also remember to say how surprised I was this year to find out that my Navy-trained electronics technician husband could not figure out the wires in a circuit and told me that he did not have to shut off the power to change a light switch! David is so good at fixing things I almost believed him, but I knew better and shut off the breaker myself. In fact, to my surprise, I figured out how to rewire the whole switch myself. Well, I had no choice. David just couldn't seem to do it.

I should remember to say how surprised I was only a few months ago that the person who could analyze and fix just about any problem, could not solve a water leak. We had water puddling all over the kitchen floor at times. David looked and looked for the leak. Finally he told me that he would have to rip out the wall behind the sink to replace the trap under the sink. He told me that is the place where the metal in a water pipe wears out. It's where the pipe turns in a "U". A weak spot.

Rip out the wall? This sounded doubtful to me. It was dry under the sink. I remarked that we had been married for over 30 years and had never had a pipe fail in such a spot before! I decided to look myself and, within a few minutes, spotted a pinhole spray of water coming from the rubber hose to the washing machine, not ten feet away from the kitchen sink. The repair took no time at all. How could he have missed this?

I should remember to say that David never (absolutely never) initiates the idea to go out to do anything together anymore, even out to dinner or to the movies. He will talk about what we should do, but then never take any step toward actually doing it. I'm the initiator, and I am so, so sick of being the initiator. When we go, David really enjoys it and always says that we should do it more often, but he never thinks about planning anything. No social event seems to draw his attention or interest.

I should remember to say that David seems so distant and weird sometimes. He assumes that everyone wants his big black lab to jump up on them as they walk, jog or run down the street in the opposite direction. People back away and try to get away but still David stops, starts talking, lets the dog hang loose enough to run to the person and jump on him or her He thinks it's fine. I tell him not to do it and he gets angry with me. He walks the dogs through neighbors' driveways and front yards. One lady came out of her house and yelled at him. Last year, he cleared out a lot of old tree limbs from our yard and put them in our neighbor's woods. When I asked him about it, he thought it was okay. Our neighbor has now put up big orange "No Trespassing" signs.

I should remember to say that David is scared or uneasy about small things like finding the bathroom in a restaurant. One time, he left me sitting in a movie theater alone 15 minutes after we arrived. He was coughing and left the theater, presumably just to get a drink of water. But he never came back. Instead, he went out to the car and sat there, leaving me all alone in the theater. Later, he said he did not return to his seat because he did not want to bother anyone in the theater. He got very angry with me for my being angry about being left alone in the theater for two hours. He seemed to think this was okay and I shouldn't be upset.

I am having trouble surviving his version of normal. He is like a living robot. Someone who breathes, but doesn't think or feel or plan or get excited about anything. The weird things just go on and on, and as I start to really think about them, I am shocked at myself for not having put it all together much earlier. Whatever has happened to David has happened to me as well. It crept up so slowly and so quietly that it was suddenly all there before both of us.

One of the craziest things I should remember to say is that David lost his truck a year ago. This was really the first significant thing that happened that got me thinking that indeed, something big-time is wrong here. He had driven his black truck from his work building to Town Hall, which was about a mile away. At the same time, David's boss drove the blue work truck to Town Hall. After completing his business at Town Hall, David got into the wrong truck. He climbed into the blue work truck and drove it back to his building, leaving his black truck behind in the Town Hall parking lot.

This left David's boss stranded at the Town Hall parking lot and it left David convinced that someone had stolen his truck from his work building parking lot. He was so convinced that he called the police. It was left to me to set things right, to figure out what had happened, to leave my job and to get the respective trucks back to their rightful places. I somehow explained it to his boss too.

David, of course, had joked about how funny this all was. I had to admit it was funny, but it was also strange business. It was the first of many times that I was left to pick up the pieces, making it right for David because he just couldn't keep things straight.

I should remember to mention all the lists that David writes, the pens and pencils he hoards in his drawer, the rituals he has adopted for dish washing or pet feeding. I should remember to say that David made quiche without the eggs and coffee without the coffeepot.

I should remember to say that it finally dawned on me why David spreads out the newspaper on the table at night before he goes to bed. It's to try to memorize the date. Oh my. Why didn't I figure this out a long time ago? He doesn't know what day it is!

I don't like putting this together, taking such small or temporary things and painting a picture like this. It doesn't feel right. I feel like I am ratting David out. It feels like I am his enemy, not his partner. Yet, why have I not done this before? Why have I been avoiding this need to step back and look at it all, honestly and openly?

I should remember to say that I have a husband I no longer know.

✦ ✦ ✦ ✦ ✦ ✦

It's almost April. David had the brain scan and we received the report that said that it was normal for an adult at his age. Now I was feeling a bit of anger at not having a medical reason for all of this weirdness. For most of the day, I wondered if that meant that David is normal and this is all in my head. I'm complaining over nothing at all.

But then I got on the Internet and found that there is a lot more that needs exploring. This could be partially depression- or alcohol-induced loss of brain cells/brain functioning. Although David no longer drinks, over a five-year period he did drink a lot. He really was very depressed then. Maybe he still is. He could certainly have killed off lots of brain cells during that time. Maybe it's a hidden tumor? He has no sense of smell. Where are the olfactory lobes? I'll have to look that up. It might not be early Alzheimer's Disease. Wouldn't that have shown up on the MRI?

David's response to the MRI news was that his memory problems are caused by the fact that he has such long lists. There are his kitchen lists, his workshop lists, and then I add a long list of things for him to do. That's why he forgets things on the list. I told him that the things he feels so burdened by are the things of normal daily living, no different from anyone else. Forgetting something from one of his many lists is not a concern. What is a concern is that when I say something, two minutes later he does not remember it. When we have a conversation, two minutes later we never had it. The lists upon lists are building into such a jumbled series of things to remember that he is creating his own problems. He is scatterbrained. That concerns me. Is being scatterbrained an illness? We have to wait for the neuropsych appointment. It's scheduled for May.

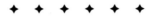

As we ease into early spring, David's mood and patterns don't change much. When I left for work this morning, David asked me what I wanted for dinner. I said, "Hmmm, steak would be good." He agreed. I got home to find a new package of hot dogs on the counter. I told David, "No, I said no more hot dogs. We are having them twice a week or more because you keep buying hot dogs!" I can say this in a way that angers David or in a way that is more good-humored. It's always an extra effort, but I choose the latter. So, David is not angry and he goes to the refrigerator and starts rummaging around to see if we have something else. No, he doesn't find anything.

I say, "That's okay, go ahead with the hot dogs, only please don't fry them. I cannot eat another fried hot dog. Boil them or steam them or broil them, whatever. Just not fried."

"Oh yes," David says. "Okay, I'll boil them."

So, I leave the kitchen to get changed. In a few minutes, David comes in with a small bag containing six frozen chicken tenders from the freezer. He asks if I think it's enough for dinner.

I say, "David, we decided that you would make the hot dogs. You were going to boil the hot dogs."

Yes, well, he could make both of them, he replies. "Okay," I say. "Make both of them or, you know, you could just boil the hot dogs."

About ten minutes later, I went into the kitchen. The new package of hot dogs was nowhere in sight, the frozen chicken tenders were nowhere in sight. On the counter was a Ziploc bag with three hot dogs in it. "Where are the new hot dogs you bought?" I ask.

David looks up and says, "What hot dogs? Oh, I don't know. Where did they go? Maybe I put them away." He goes to the refrigerator and finds the new package in there. "But I found these (the three orphan hot dogs) and they're older so we should use these. Are they enough?"

I open the bag and they smell awful. "Three days," I say. "Meat only lasts three days in the refrigerator."

David says, "I don't understand why meat goes bad so fast in the refrigerator."

I ignore his ignorance. "Okay, so you are going to cook the new hot dogs?" I ask.

"Yes," David says.

"You're going to boil them, right?"

"Right," David says as he points to the saucepan (not the frying pan). "That's as big a pot as I've got, but it will do."

"Okay," I say and leave the kitchen.

Twenty minutes later, David calls me for dinner. I come into the kitchen and there are five *fried* hot dogs waiting in the frying pan!

And so it goes.

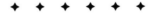

It's now late April and David has been back at work for about three weeks. His spirits have started to lift noticeably. He is in a better mood. He is more focused, but still sometimes drifty. He still wanders around the kitchen trying to look busy. At times he can't seem to apply himself to anything other than going to work and coming home, but then his work routine has just started up again.

There are now good days and bad days. This is a bad day. David is off tonight. I could tell almost as soon as I got home. He was quieter, moodier. I asked if he wanted to take the dogs for a walk. He said, "Yeah, I guess so," but was not at all pleased or happy about it.

I told him that he had an appointment coming up soon with the neuropsychologist. He wanted to know why and seemed disgusted. He said he thought he was all done. What was this about? I reminded him that there were two follow-ups ordered by his neurologist—some blood work and this testing appointment. David said that he already got the blood work done and this was a psychologist appointment—he didn't need a psychologist. I tried to explain that this is a specially trained psychologist—a scientist, not a counselor. The testing will be quite thorough, lasting nearly the whole day.

During the walk, he kept questioning my handling of my dog in a critical sort of way. Why did I pull the dog back just then? Do I think the dog understands English? I walked on ahead of David and he mostly kept slightly behind me. I'm sad that it is such a beautiful early evening and David is grumpy, disinterested and sullen.

It was already 7:00 p.m. when we got back but still light enough for me to spot check my bulbs in the back yard. I could see David walking across the kitchen several times, stopping, walking back. He wasn't really doing anything, except maybe waiting for me to come inside. The cat hadn't eaten. I came inside and fed the cat. There was no food for us. I started to cook. David hovered around me, watching what I was doing. After I put some food in the oven, David sat at the kitchen table. He wasn't really waiting for dinner, just sitting. He has not thought about dinner or eating. He has shown no interest in it whatsoever. I think I have to just forget that dinner is a joint venture. Dinner is now something that I want and need when I come home, but something that David has absolutely no thought about or interest in.

What is he interested in? Anything?

I'm now wondering if he is eating any lunch. It's just dawned on me that he has not been making his lunches for work and this is his third week back. That is unusual. When I ask him, he says that he has been going to Wendy's for the past three weeks for lunch. He gets the same thing each time, 15 days in a row now: a spicy chicken meal and a Frosty. He says he is getting tired of it, but he just hasn't had time to go to the store to get things for lunch. That's why he keeps eating the same thing for lunch every day.

I don't think that's what's going on. I have an impending sense of dread that I just can't shake.

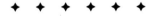

So here it is June already. The appointment for a neuropsych exam has come and gone and so has an interminable wait for the results, the written report. The doctor was good enough to call me in advance and share the results and her thoughts and her prognosis and her advice. Of course, I needed none of it. I needed absolutely nothing more to tell me what was wrong than what I had seen and heard and experienced so far.

I was quite sure what we were dealing with. The idea of a diagnosis or something to call it seemed a bit strange and foreign. Later, it became more significant. The number of times that I would have to refer back to it became too numerous to count. "When was he diagnosed?" "What a shame. How long ago was he diagnosed?" "Where was he diagnosed?" "Who diagnosed him?" "How old was he when he was diagnosed?" How little I knew then about the importance in time of such a moment!

At least to others. It was never important to me. Frosting on the cake, so to speak. Not necessary for me really, but necessary to the medical community and the caregiving community. A way to judge his progress through this debilitating illness. I'm not as bitter now as I was then and I'm not as angry now as I was then, but it is ever so difficult to go back to those days and feel what I was feeling then. Like my world was being invaded by people who had no business being in it. Like David's dignity was being put on a milepost for everyone to gawk at.

Our neuropsychologist was a wonderful woman who asked questions in a gentle and supportive and comforting manner. I talked and talked as though released from all the hostilities I had been feeling toward David. I told her about all of David's shortcomings with gusto. I laughed with her over some of the craziness. David laughed with her as well and often seemed to take on a childlike giddiness and distraction, which she captured in her observations.

David's verbal comprehension abilities were quite good. He had no difficulties with speech or writing. I learned about Working Memory and Processing Speed, categories in which

David scored quite low. Then we got to memory and learning. "Memory and learning testing demonstrate severe impairment."

In General Memory and a few other categories, David actually scored a negative percentile. I'm not sure how that's possible. Everything listed that had the word "memory" also had the attached description, "Extremely Low" in terms of his performance. "His poor memory performance would be expected to lead to functional difficulties in daily living... there are severe impairments in memory and learning and in executive functioning."

"Significant frontal system dysfunction."

"Severe impairments in memory and learning consistent with an Alzheimer's Dementia."

"A frontal variant of Alzheimer's Disease with severe memory loss and frontal features."

My first thought was for me. I felt such relief to know that, in fact, there was really something wrong. It was not in my imagination. Although I felt guilty about thinking of myself first, I was so glad to know that I was validated in my observations and that I was not the root cause of all of David's problems as he so often tried to tell me.

And yet, within a nanosecond, I felt the looming dread of what was ahead of both of us as this was not only David's disease. It belonged to both of us, and we would have to face it together.

I asked, "So, what are we talking about... ahh... you know, what are we talking about in terms of David's ahhh... future? You can be direct. I think I know what this means."

She responded in a forthright manner as I had requested. Still, it was hard to take.

"Seven years. I'm sorry, but that is his life expectancy. When it strikes early like this, it can be very fast. I would say that seven years is about right, given what we know about this."

I felt like a wet blanket had been wrapped around my head. I could not hear any more. I could barely breathe, and I could barely carry the weight of my head on my shoulders. It was so evident and yet so secretive at the same time. I was most appreciative of her manner, her directness with me, her willingness to talk at length on the phone with me about David and what to expect in the years ahead. She knew this was earth-shattering, explosive, mind-altering stuff, and she knew that I desperately needed to know all of it. This is not something I could share with our daughters just yet. They will need to absorb this slowly.

When the seven-page report arrived in the mail, I left it on the kitchen table for David to read, but he never read it. So, I told David the results while we were out walking the dogs on yet another golden late spring afternoon, an afternoon with the lilacs now in full bloom and the root smell of sweet earth rising from the ground. David's reaction was as mildly disaffected as I seemed to sound to myself in telling him about it. Our silence confirmed that we had already known what was coming, and it was obvious that we just didn't need to verbalize this. We never looked at each other. We focused on our dogs, the late spring sunlight and the winding country lane where we liked to walk each day.

We had had plenty of years together. This was not really going to change a thing for us, and yet, we knew that it would affect our lives. It is a devastating illness for old people. What is it like for relatively young people? We will just take it as it comes, day by day.

We'll just do the best that we can for as long as we can.

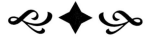

Getting married was not on my radar screen when I first met David. In fact, I had dated very little in high school and I was eagerly looking forward to my first year of college at Smith, which was mostly an all-girls school. Boyfriends were certainly not on my mind. Yet, three days after I graduated from high school, there he was, looking at me from across the room with a big Texas smile. This was my blind date for the evening. He was skinny, with a long thin face, bushy eyebrows, brown hair and intense green eyes that were so expressive that they seemed to dance every time he smiled.

We were supposed to actually go somewhere that night. As it turned out, we drove out to Provincetown at the tip of the Cape with another couple, and David and I never got out of the car. We sat together in the back seat and talked and kissed and talked and kissed. It was as though I had always known him, or had always known that one day he would find me from across a room. It was just a matter of time.

Two weeks later at Paine's Creek in Brewster, David asked me to marry him and I said yes. We had a few more weekends together and then I barely saw him over the next seven months. David was in the Navy. He shipped out to California and from there was sent on a Westpac cruise that included Vietnam. After returning to California, he immediately took leave, making his way back across the United States by train and bus. He walked into the Smith College library in full dress blues and kissed me on the back of my neck as I sat in a study carrel. It was like a scene from *An Officer and a Gentleman*. He swept me away. My friends at school were quite impressed.

I managed to finish my first year of college while David was sent back out to sea. He was cruising the Mekong Delta while I participated in sit-ins and demonstrations both on and off campus. We never had final exams that year. There were too many Smith College students over at Brown and Amherst and the University of Massachusetts protesting the war. All I knew was that I wanted David home, safe and sound.

He did come home for our wedding the following December, and then I joined him in California. It was an exciting time. War news still had us on our toes and then there was the 1971 earthquake. David was out on a three-week deployment at the time, while I was in our little apartment in Long Beach. The men were not told about the earthquake at home until they came into port two weeks later. The Pacific fleet did not have laptops or Internet communications back then. We just had to wait it out. I survived some bricks flying off the walls and also the apartment complex swimming pool unfilling itself through mini-tidal waves as the earth shook.

We developed a routine. When David was in port and got paid, we would buy our groceries at the commissary, go out to eat and then wait for the next paycheck. In between, we went window shopping and rode our bicycles. I returned to school, attending the local junior college. Our life was simple, but we had fun. With David, nothing was ever very serious except laughing and having fun. That was the order of the day. In fact, David's motto seemed to be "Carpe diem." At the time, I thought sometimes that he was foolish and immature. Now I look back and think,

Good that we had fun back then. Good that David balanced out my serious side. Without his enthusiasm and positive attitude, I'm not sure I would have been a very good partner over the many long years of our marriage.

We were very well balanced together. His fun-loving spirit balanced out my constant need to worry to excess about things, to be a stressful overachiever.

✦ ✦ ✦ ✦ ✦ ✦

Following David's diagnosis, the summer progresses with David working and appearing to be more functional. It seems that work is certainly a boost to his energy level. I'm glad to see him smiling again and telling me about the luxury yachts that he visits each day with his harbormaster pumpout boat. David's job is to pump out septic holding tanks on these boats. It would be a job that another person would love to hate, but not David. With a smile and a wave, he greets the boaters, accomplishes the task, exchanges news.

We are into a season of minor irritations. They do make me impatient, but really, that's about it. I have to step back every once in a while to sum it all up and remember that this is really not that bad, at least not right now.

There are interesting things, like the salt. I was looking everywhere for the salt. For two days I looked for the salt. David noticed my frustration. "What on earth are you looking for?" he asked.

"I'm looking for the salt. I haven't had a grain of salt in two days because I can't find it anywhere," I replied.

"Well, that's because you probably put it somewhere illogical."

Ahh no, that would be you, not me, I thought to myself. *How can he take on this superior attitude with me when he is the one with memory problems?* Then suddenly he asked, "Did you look in the refrigerator?"

I laughed and said, "No, of course not! But I've looked through all the cabinets at least ten times."

At that point, David got up and walked over to the refrigerator. He reached in toward the back of one of the shelves and pulled out the salt, bringing it triumphantly over to the table.

"How did you know that it was in there?" I asked with an astonished look on my face.

"I don't know," he replied.

"But you must have known somehow, subconsciously, that you put the salt in the refrigerator?"

"No, really, I don't know. I just knew it was there."

We both laughed over this. Of course, it was logical that a person with Alzheimer's Disease might put the salt in the refrigerator, so I should have looked there. Still, how is it possible that he had no memory of putting the salt in there, yet he knew where it was? Weird. Very weird.

So, the salt has disappeared a few times since then. The pepper is on the opposite counter from where it usually sits, now being unwilling to return home without its partner. We are into disorganization. There are books and papers on the table and on the cabinet, along with screws and pens and notes and batteries.

David makes the same comments to me over and over and over. There are themes like the water theme. He must drink a lot of water. It is really important that he drink a lot of water. Or the ice theme. The ice in the cooler he takes to work has not melted. Do I know why? Well, it has nothing to do with the quality of the cooler, David tells me, it has to do with how often it's opened. Did I know that? If you don't open the cooler all day, there will still be ice in there the next morning. Oh, how he loves to lecture me! I haven't tried the ultimate cooler test, but it's a cooler barely bigger than a lunch box. Somehow, I doubt that the ice cubes in it will last 24 hours in this summer heat wave unless we park the whole cooler in the freezer.

Then there are the poplar trees. It seems that they are ready to fall over. We see them everywhere while we walk the dogs together. David has catalogued many trees in people's yards that he is concerned about, and so he carefully watches them each time we walk by. He exclaims, "See that one? It's going to be next. How awful. These poor people. I hope it doesn't damage their house." He could sell lottery tickets! People could guess when each tree is going to fall over. For David, it's not a question of if, but when. With great seriousness and certainty, he worries obsessively about these trees falling over.

How we walk, on which side of the street and in what direction is now starting to be a theme and a problem. He still walks faster than I do, but he does not like walking with his back to the cars. "Why do these people come to Cape Cod only to speed down the road? Where do they have to get to so fast? Those people don't like dogs if they are so careless about driving. Look how that car almost hit us!"

Then it's the weather and David's miserable perspective. "This has been the most awful summer. The weather has been awful. Not one really warm day so far." I keep contradicting him, saying that it's just not so. It has been incredibly hot and muggy for over a month. We have had nothing but beautiful sunshine for almost two months. How can he think that this has been an awful summer?

✦ ✦ ✦ ✦ ✦ ✦

Small victories are so labor intensive that it's exhausting. It took seven hours to put a new gas grill together. I actually thought that this was a project that David could handle. The instructions had no words, only pictures with arrows and photos and actual-sized screw patterns.

When I came home from the store and saw all the pieces all over the driveway and David's obvious confusion, I knew right away that I had to give up what I was doing to help him through it. It was aggravating and excruciating to watch him ponder over each picture and part, then forget where he was and re-ponder the same part. He was able to do some parts of it on his own. That was encouraging, but when it came to the most simple things, like finding nuts to fit the screws for which they had not provided enough nuts, that was a big problem. I sent David back to the workshop. We have so many nuts. We have to have the right ones.

He came out of the workshop with a large box of nuts, saying he could not find any that would fit. I took three off the top that I thought might fit. Two out of these three turned out to be a perfect fit. So I thought, *How can David look at a problem like this and find it so impossible?* This one seemed so clear to me. A huge box of nuts, so many that it would have been literally impossible that we would not have at least twenty of every conceivable size. This is simple, just pick one out and try it. He found the box, but he cannot take one nut out of the box to see if it fits?

It's part of my nature to analyze everything ad nauseum. But I also have a need to understand what is happening to David. How can it be so clear and yet so impossible to him? Was it the number of nuts in the box that overwhelmed him? That must be it. I have to reduce his choices. I have to create successes for him. He feels so good when he can actually do something, solve a problem. I want him to feel good, but I have to lay it all out like a preschool activity. It's frustrating.

During the early years of our marriage, we had very little money. It was up to David to fix whatever broke or didn't work right. From plumbing to electrical work, to car repairs, to woodworking and building, there was nothing he couldn't do. I would worry sometimes when he had our VW bus in 300 pieces spread out over the garage floor, but he always managed to get it back together and get us back on the road. I can remember times when we would take a drive out to the country, for lack of any money to do something more exotic. The bus would break down, and there he would be under the bus in the middle of nowhere with rags and pieces of metal and tape, making it work again. Forcing it to work again. He'd jump back in the driver's seat with a big smile and we were off again.

Incongruous now that he cannot fit a nut to a screw. I want to run into the bathroom and cry or throw up, I'm not sure which one it will be until I get there.

I have been on vacation this week, but it hasn't felt like a vacation. With the extra time taken to attend to these matters that stump David more and more often, I am finding it difficult to relax. I am on the alert for the next problem, trading one set of frustrations for another. When I do go back to work next week, it will be another complexity of frustrations that will have me constantly stretched. Not stretched to the limit, though. I can't be stretched to the limit because I do know that there is so much more ahead that I will have to be ready to handle.

✦　✦　✦　✦　✦　✦

We are into September, and David has been on Aricept for about four weeks now. His neurologist prescribed this medication as the best choice out of three that he reviewed for us. It will not cure David for sure, but it is supposed to help him maintain his current skill levels for a while longer—perhaps six months longer than would otherwise be the case, maybe a year longer. For mid and late stage, we just don't know. The research is lacking. But at this stage, the data is pretty good. It should help.

David can remember to take these pills. I find that odd. My analytic side wants to know why. He has only missed one. Of course, it's very important to him to find a cure or anything that will help, so he does focus on taking his pills. It is just weird to me that if he can focus on taking his pills because they are so important, why aren't other things at least as important to remember?

Unfortunately, though, in my opinion the pills have not made the slightest difference. If anything, he is worse. I think this is progressing fast. He absolutely must go to the grocery store on each of his days off, and so I now have two eight-cone packages of Nutty-Buddies. I like them, but 16 is more than I would eat in a year. We have so many boxes of dog bones and varieties of dog treats that the dogs really don't need dog food any more. When he was off to the store again, I told him I had enough dinners on hand, but he went anyway and bought chicken and pork chops. We have to hurry up to eat these things before they go bad, or I have to stop what I am doing to rewrap and freeze them for later. Somehow, these things always circle back to me and eat up my time.

One day, David saw that I had bought broccoli. That gave him an idea to look up broccoli recipes. Now, David used to be a great cook. It was always fun to come to dinner when David cooked, because he would try new things and actually use a cookbook, whereas I was a meat-loaf-and-potatoes kind of cook. Very standard and very unimaginative. So, he found a recipe he liked with cream and Gruyere cheese and called me at work to tell me about it. It sounded great! But when I got home that night, he said that he was too harried to make the recipe after all. No problem. I had leftovers and could make a salad.

But now in the refrigerator, there are two huge new bunches of broccoli, Gruyere cheese and a pint of cream. What will I do with these things?

Should I hide the ingredients so he forgets about this project, so it won't bother him? Or should I just cook it up? But then if I do that, will he get mad at me for interfering? Why do I let his problems become my problems?

✦   ✦   ✦   ✦   ✦   ✦

David is blaming me a lot lately and I absolutely revolt against that, so that we now get into shouting matches. He forgets them after a while, but I don't. He says I made him sell the boat. That's not true. The boat continues to sit in the yard. A friend wants to buy it and we have had several discussions so far, but nothing else. David apparently doesn't want to talk about it. So, the boat continues to sit in the yard.

The workshop is my fault. How? I planned it and built it to hold David's many wood and boat projects, as well as shop tools we had inherited through the years. It is a beautiful building, but now a complete mess inside. I have no time to go in there and sort out things that I do not understand. Metal parts, wood parts, odd screws, large and small tools, tubes of putty, boat ropes, things of that sort. David cannot or will not do it. He just seems to have totally lost interest in anything outside the kitchen. He tells me he cannot work out there in the cold, but it has not been cold for five months.

I can't help feeling that the things that he wants to do are girl-things. He wants to be a girl. He wants to wash dishes all day and all night. He wants to wash and fold the clothes. He wants to go to the grocery store. He wants to wash the kitchen floor. He wants to vacuum the kitchen floor. Why doesn't he want to sweep out the shop, sort out the junk, organize all the boat stuff, take trash to the dump? What about gluing that chair with the loose rungs, fixing the broken dog fence, mowing and raking the yard? Of course, my expectations of him are unrealistic, but in my own way, I think I can ward off the inevitable by continuing to expect so much of him.

✦ ✦ ✦ ✦ ✦ ✦

Back on winter layoff.

David wonders why there are so many coffee cups in the sink waiting to be washed. Last night, I tried to show him. "David, you take out a cup, fill it with coffee and put it in the microwave and forget about it. Then you make a new pot of coffee. You fill a new cup and bring it over to the counter and forget about it. Then you fill another new cup and bring it to the table. You then think that must be my cup so you get another new cup and bring that to the table as well."

Why do I bother? He does the same thing with cat food dishes. They are everywhere. We only have one cat, but he puts cat dishes in the dining room and on the kitchen counter and out on the picnic table outside and under the boat outside and in the workshop where we have a cat door. Then it hits me. He installed that cat door only last year! Only last year, he was able to install a cat door! It's unfathomable to think of him doing such a project this year.

That's how much he has changed and in so little time. This sets me up for the whole day wondering and worrying about our future. *What will he be like in another year?*

David is more and more negative and that has me upset as well. The themes continue, particularly the awful weather theme. Yet our warm and sunny summer has continued into a lusciously beautiful fall. He says that's not true. It's been cold. He is tired of being cold.

He is tired, tired, tired. Always complains of being tired. He sighs a lot and groans a lot. Lately he has been holding onto me in the mornings, saying that he does not want us to get out of bed. That would be nice except that when he gets out of bed, he has no interest in anything other than being negative and critical.

Mostly, I am angry. David used to be a sounding board. Now I not only do not have a partner, I do not have a sounding board. In half an hour, I will meet with the fifth contractor coming to give me a price on installing a new gas furnace and water heater. I have learned all about venting natural gas and how the stove and furnace have to be on separate vents. How if it exhausts through the chimney, the chimney has to be lined, and if it exhausts through a vent pipe, that pipe has to be three feet away from any window, door, corner, or ell of the house. It is illegal to have both LP gas and natural gas in one residence, so the current stove either has to go or it has to be converted. I now have the 800 number to GE so I can call to see if I can order the conversion parts. My local supplier was not a bit helpful.

I do this in my spare time with no help whatsoever from David.

I'm angry.

I have started to tell these contractor people that I deal with that they are not to speak to David: "My husband has some memory problems, and he will be unable to record a message from you or to discuss your proposal, so please make sure that you get through to me personally." I give them my cell number for good measure just to make sure that I will actually get their messages. David will invariably lose any message left on our home phone.

I'm finding that it's becoming necessary to be nasty and devious.

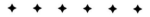

I am surprised that my last entry was so angry.

More recently, I've thought that the Aricept was having a positive effect after all, since David seems to be a little more focused and tuned in, a little sharper. It's November now and he has been on it for several months. Well, a little sharper also makes him a little more difficult to get along with. He is snappy. He makes remarks, and retorts, and angry little snappy comments more than he used to. I have blamed that on the Aricept. If, indeed, what I am seeing is that he is more aware, then he is more aware of his own illness and it is making him angrier. It makes sense.

Who would want to have to deal with this insidious disease invading every part of your life?

Stupid things like today. He had the TV on in the kitchen. I came in and started to watch a story about a family divorce and child support situation that had gone all the way to the Supreme Court. The father wasn't the biological father of the three sons for whom he was forced to pay child support. Meanwhile, David goes on and on about the historical significance of his Little Debbie doll. Okay, I ordered the doll for Christmas because David likes Little Debbie snack cakes. Part of his fun-loving nature. He has always loved Little Debbies and when he saw this doll, well, he had to have it. It's a Barbie doll with a shopping bag full of little cardboard-boxed Little Debbie snack cakes. David loves it. But we lost her shoes, so she will never be a pricey artifact 100 years from now. But David does not buy that. He will not throw the box away that she came in. He is going on and on about how much money she will be worth.

When he notices that I am paying attention to the TV and not to him, he says, "Fine, that show is obviously more important than I am." Snap, snap. Well, I just cannot listen to him drone on about stupid things. He had the TV on in the first place. I just happened to walk into the kitchen and started to watch it. So, I reply, "Fine, and you can watch the TV without me in the room." I then get my coffee and leave the kitchen. So it goes.

It is hard living with someone who has absolutely no thought or care about you whatsoever. I was looking for consolation because I had to have a tooth pulled after just spending $850 on it. "Oh, that's too bad," says David. "Well, it will be over before you know it." He did not ask when it would be. When my appointment was cancelled one hour before the extraction, I did not bother telling him about it. It would have been empty conversation. He would not have remembered that I was going to have a tooth pulled, that the appointment was cancelled, that the appointment was rescheduled. He would not have been able to understand my emotional roller coaster or to sympathize with me in any meaningful way. So, I will build up my emotional armor for this next appointment all over again... alone.

We saw the neurologist yesterday. This time, David could spell WORLD backwards, but he could not remember the three things that the doctor asked him to remember and tell him later. He also did not know what day of the week it was. I nearly burst out laughing. Then, he did not know what month it was. He said it was September. This time, I really had to fight for control not to burst out laughing. I would have been so embarrassed for us both if I had laughed, but we probably would have both burst out laughing at the same time if we looked at each other. I really just wanted to turn to him and give him a little hint, but I just stared straight ahead and held my breath. The doctor then said that he'd better do some of the tests again—the reflex pokes and the follow-my-commands tests. I sat in the chair in his office while he took David into the other room.

"Well, I do see a decline." The doctor summed it up as he re-entered his office. He seemed a bit stumped. "In just this short time, a decline. Well, I will need him back here in four months and if there is further decline, we will just have to see about switching him to something else, because we are not going to *not* be aggressive about this at his age and this does not seem to be working, but we will be able to tell that at his next appointment.

No, we cannot *not* treat this aggressively."

David's doctor has such a negative bedside manner that it is amazing that he is allowed to practice medicine on real patients, particularly those with family members. He is a nerdy smart doctor with no people skills at all and practices almost 100 percent skepticism regarding all manner of things we have lightly conversed about so far. But David seems to like him. This doctor was so absolutely sold on Aricept—"really the only choice for David, the only medication with solid research behind it for treatment at this stage of the disease." Now I saw surprise in his face. Now we have stumped the nerdy little scientist at his own game. In truth, he is a very smart and knowledgeable neurologist. Top of his game. So what's next for us? What's next if a good doctor prescribes good medicine and it does no good?

So, okay, David is declining and what am I doing about it? I tried to apply for long-term-care insurance but there it was: Question 6—"Do you have Alzheimer's or some brain syndrome or dementia?" It seems that these terms are automatic disqualifiers, but if we just say David has "memory problems," that may not be an automatic disqualifier. Interesting. I called his doctor's office. What is David's actual diagnosis? It may seem strange, but no one had actually said the words to me other than in the initial report from his neuropsych exam that said, "probable Alzheimer's Disease with a frontal variant." I really did not know if that stuck. I was hoping, of course, that it had not stuck, that we were not stuck with this disease.

The answer was immediate with just a hint of surprise at my question. "Alzheimer's." Surprise on me. So, with that one word, no long-term-care insurance for us. Now what's next?

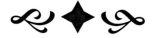

David's world is not illogical. It is warped. I wanted to go out to Provincetown and decided my day off today would be a good day to go. David immediately started to pull out his long underwear and examine his jeans to find the warmest, sturdiest pair. He does not want to be cold. He remembers P'town as cold and blustery, so he wants to be prepared. Only, it's 52 degrees out today. Late November and 52 degrees. A gift, a lovely warm fall day. I tell David that it's warm out and he won't need the long underwear. It does not change his mind. He pulls them on. "I want to be warm," he says. Oddly enough, he does not sweat throughout the day. I am wearing a light jacket and he is in three layers, but he does not sweat.

I can recall lots of cold days when I would be the one running back to the house for a warmer jacket or a sweatshirt to put on under my jacket. David would be in a T-shirt and feeling no cold whatsoever. Now our roles seem reversed. He is always cold and I seem to be always warm. Maybe for me, it's the energy it takes to watch over David that is keeping me warm. We have a nice outing in P'town with a wonderful fish chowder lunch. It's what I've needed. A break. Just a little chance to get away. David enjoys the trip immensely. We look out over the harbor together.

We have a picture from this harbor taken over 30 years ago. We were between California and our newly assigned duty station in Hawaii, on a return trip home to Cape Cod to visit my parents. Very rarely, there would be a pleasure trip in my father's old Chris Craft, which he kept in Sesuit Harbor in Dennis. Besides being a scientist, my father was a serious fisherman, filling up the freezer each year with flounder. So, it wasn't often that he would take us out on his boat just to enjoy the water. But on this day he did. My mother and I packed up a cooler with sandwiches, and we motored out across Cape Cod Bay, David and I stretched out on the bow, arriving in P'town just in time for lunch.

We ate our sandwiches and drank beers, looking out over this same harbor. A large tuna had been brought in that day and lots of people were taking pictures. My parents loved David. My father was always talking to him about things technical and electronic. My mother would dance and laugh and sing with him. I found myself feeling sad that they were no longer with us, but glad that they only ever knew the old David, the David who was never sick.

✦ ✦ ✦ ✦ ✦ ✦

The trees-falling-down theme continues. Every time we walk, without fail, David comments about the trees falling down. So many trees falling down. He chuckles like it is a big joke.

There is a beautiful stone foundation supporting a raised driveway that we pass each day on our walk. Each time we pass it, David comments that the people should do something about it. It is "pooching" out in the middle so it is falling apart. "They should fix it before it falls apart," David keeps saying.

Well, one day, maybe 10 years from now, some of the rocks will actually fall out and the driveway will start to crumble. David is not wrong. It's just a question of when. Still, he has assumed an occupation of worrying about it and commenting about it, and he is convinced that its ultimate fate is imminent. What a shame that those people are just letting it happen!

I continue to wonder if David thinks it is a shame that the house paint is peeling and that he did nothing to fix it or that the leaves have yet to be raked up and he has not picked up a rake. Or that the workshop is still a gigantic junk pile inside and he will not clean it. It is warped, selective worrying.

When we walk, David sometimes veers off our normal path as he walks with Annie, his black lab. He says that it's Annie who wants to go in these off-directions. Well, it's David who is holding the leash. He veers off into people's driveways and across their property. I keep telling him to stay on the street, but he jeers at me, telling me I am always criticizing him.

Maybe he's right. Maybe I am. Is it my imagination or is David walking slower? I seem to have no trouble keeping up with him now. He stops to stare at things or to comment. It makes our walks so long and slow sometimes now. I need regular exercise, but I don't feel like I'm getting it this way.

✦ ✦ ✦ ✦ ✦ ✦

We have gone out twice in our dress-up clothes recently. It's not something you do too often on Cape Cod. Once, it was to visit Kristin's future mother-in-law on Thanksgiving. Kristin is getting married in April! Her husband-to-be is a fisherman and does construction on the side. His family lives about 10 miles away and so we are going to meet them for the first time.

I gave David 24 hours' notice that he would have to make sure that he had clothes ready to go, and then I reminded him again at least 10 times throughout Thanksgiving morning. I was not particularly worried, because David left the kitchen to ready his clothes and returned, telling me his clothes were all ready.

About 15 minutes before it was time to leave, David was frantic that his pants did not fit. By about four years and four inches they did not fit! He had picked out some old dress pants. There were *no* other pants to be had. I didn't realize that he had gained several pounds after quitting smoking about a year ago. Somewhere, there was a pair of dress khakis that would surely still fit, but they were nowhere to be found. Finally, Lisa and I found them in the laundry, pulled them out, and she ironed them while he concentrated on his upper half.

I ask him why he does not buy another pair of pants. He replies that he has been told not to buy things, implying, of course, that it's my fault. His dresser and closet are a circus of old, musty-smelling, too-small clothes that he does not seem to be able to clean up. He may go through them and fold them up, but never will part with a single thing. The more he has, the more it confuses him.

I'm not sure why I didn't realize that this was quickly becoming too much for him. Probably because a man's closet is his castle or something like that. I felt that I would be infringing on his personal space to interfere with his closet or his dresser. But now, I am determined to buy him new clothes for Christmas and literally throw out half of what he has accumulated. This is my job now and I should have realized it a lot earlier.

A few weeks later, we were getting ready to go out to the symphony and, like a repeat performance, there was David with no shirt to wear. I had reminded him repeatedly throughout the day that he would need to get his clothes ready, and he had said that he was all ready. At 10 minutes before time to go, he was frantic that he had no shirt. I very regretfully handed over the new white button-down dress shirt that I had bought him for Christmas.

David then put on a jacket that looked like it could fit a first grader.

"You can't wear that! It's way too small," I told him.

"No, it isn't. It's just fine. It's my favorite jacket." David was right. This was his favorite blue wool jacket, and we had spent a lot of money on it, but there it was. Too small. Nothing would change that.

"You have to be uncomfortable in it. You can barely even move your arms."

"Oh yes, I can. I can move my arms fine."

"No, David. This is ridiculous. You look ridiculous!"

It was like arguing with a small child. Eventually, he agreed to wear a different jacket that fit better, but what a struggle.

In my mind, I am calculating out to the future the exact number of remaining symphony performances that we will be able to attend. Very few. I love going to listen to the Cape Cod Symphony. They feed my soul. They fill my need for music and respite, delivery from the day's chores. I have bought season tickets for years.

Maybe we can continue to go through next year and then David will be too uncooperative to dress appropriately. Even if I work to organize his clothes and buy the things that he needs, it probably won't be enough. I realize I can help him only temporarily. I also realize that I am letting this all get to me in a very personal way, like it's all about me. Sometimes, it feels exactly like that. I see what's happening to us through my own life and how it impacts me, instead of being more sympathetic to David's needs.

On the way to the symphony, I noticed that David's driving seemed to be a bit jagged. He has always been a great driver. Last night, it was a little too fast and a little too jerky. He had to stop short behind a truck that was turning left. He had to ask me many times for directions or cues. Sometimes I just give them: "Turn right up here" or "We'll take the Mid-Cape Highway tonight, so turn left when you get to the stop sign." I tend to watch and wait for what he needs. He doesn't know that I do that. Maybe that is part of what is wearing me out!

✦ ✦ ✦ ✦ ✦ ✦

In his tone and his remarks, David is so mean and snappy toward me. I asked him if he could finish the dinner cooking on the stove—just spaghetti. "Just watch the spaghetti until it's done and drain it. Okay?"

"Sure," he replies.

"I'm going to take a shower," I tell him.

When I return, the spaghetti is still cooking away in the pot.

"David," I ask, totally frustrated. "Why have you left the spaghetti on the stove?"

He looks at me and he is angry. "Where have you been all this time?"

"I told you I was taking a shower," I reply.

"You left me here all this time while you take a shower? I need to take a shower too. When am I supposed to take a shower?" I tell him that my shower does not interfere with his shower. He has plenty of time to take a shower.

"Yeah, well, what about the hot water? What if you have used all the hot water?"

"No," I say. "There is plenty of hot water. I have not used all the hot water and I have not interfered with your shower."

"Have you seen my colander?" he asks.

"Yes," and I reach to take it down from a hook on the wall.

Now I realize that the missing colander was the problem. On the other counter were two old smaller colanders that David had pulled out from the cabinet. He did not want to use those. He wanted his big colander. There are only two of us. The spaghetti in the pot would barely cover the surface of a dinner plate, but he had to have his big colander. His world was falling apart for lack of the large colander and so the spaghetti would cook forever without it, but in the end, it was my shower that was the problem.

It's becoming a struggle not to enter his world and to protect my own.

Year Two

It's January. A few days ago, David had a strange episode. No doubt that it has happened before and I did not really notice, but this time it seemed very noticeable. David was a little agitated or angry. He often gets that way when he can't find something. This time, he was not looking for anything. He had a blank look. He would take a few steps in one direction, stop, seem to think and then take some steps in another direction, stop, seem to think, walk around the table, stop. I asked him several times if something was wrong. No, nothing was wrong. This lasted for at least 10 minutes or so. He had such a blank look. A little alarm bell went off in me that maybe David could have suffered a little stroke. Or, maybe this is an advance notice of what may happen in the future with more frequency.

I am going to a meeting by a local Alzheimer's agency. It's called *Alzheimer's Services of Cape Cod and the Islands*. They provide information, education and support services. I need to remember this episode and ask about it as I don't remember reading about a manifestation like this.

David is sleeping a lot. It's amazing to me how long he sleeps — anywhere from 11 to 13 hours or so. While only four or five months ago, he was periodically up in the mornings, now he is never up when I get up. He does not get up until 10 or 11 a.m. Of course, he is in the middle of his winter layoff, but this much sleeping can't be healthy. Is he depressed? Is depression part of Alzheimer's or is it all jumbled into one thing?

He has a lot of muscle jerks when he sleeps. Maybe that actually keeps him from getting a sound sleep, so that's why he needs to sleep longer. Last night, I timed the jerks. It was very steady at 10 jerks a minute or one every six seconds. At least two a minute are strong overall body jerks and the rest are smaller but seem to occur all over: upper arm, lower arm, thigh, lower leg. I realize that this is one reason that we have not been spoon sleeping. He has developed autonomous sleeping habits. We are no longer paired in anticipation of each other's changes in position as we sleep.

Anger and competitiveness rise to the surface almost every day, and we are both at fault. Today, David complained for a long time about me turning the heat up. I kept saying that it was only one degree, from 67 to 68, and for God's sake, it's January!

"You are burning me up in the kitchen!"

"Well," I reply sarcastically, "since you live in the kitchen, you have no idea how cold the rest of the house gets. I should be able to be warm in my own house."

"Well," he replies sarcastically back, "I'm the one who spends a lot of time outside, not sitting in a warm office all day like you. I'm used to the cold."

"Oh come on! You don't spend a lot of time outside. You live in the warm kitchen all the time. That's why you don't get cold."

So he thinks I just sit in an office all day. I'm so tired of him belittling what I do.

To his credit, though, he actually apologized later over the one-degree business. Well, what he said was that he couldn't remember what it was about, but he knew that he had been mean and unreasonable and he was sorry. I was quick to accept his apology and probably should have apologized back, but I didn't. He started it.

Forgetfulness also pervades our everyday lives on a constant basis. David was going to the store tonight for dog and cat food and wondered if I needed anything. I responded, "No, but..."

As though reading my mind, he finished my thought, "How about Chinese food?" he asked.

"Chinese food would be great," I replied.

We agreed that I would wait 15 minutes before ordering so he would have time to buy the dog and cat food. Over an hour later, he came home with cold Chinese food and no dog or cat food. Where had he been? Did he get lost? I'm starting to worry about him leaving the house on his own.

David could probably drive to the store blindfolded. He has been the grocery store shopper for years. I hate to go. He loves to go. I can't take this task away from him. He would think I'm crazy. Maybe I am. Maybe we both are.

✦ ✦ ✦ ✦ ✦ ✦

Tonight, I had to pick up our grandson, Devon, from his after-school program. Kris had to work late. In a rush, I left work so fast that I forgot some papers I had intended to bring home. So, I had to run back to work with Devon in tow to pick up the papers. At six o'clock, I called David to tell him that I would be late. He doesn't cook very often anymore, but I had left a canned ham and some pinto beans on the counter. He told me on the phone that he had the ham in the oven and the beans on the stove and he had cooked some corn bread. He asked me to call him back just when I was ready to leave to come home so he could warm everything up. That sounded good to me. No, that sounded too good to me to be true! It felt like old times.

At 6:30, I called David to tell him that I was leaving. It would take me about 35 minutes to get home in the snow. I dropped Devon off and when I pulled into the driveway, I noticed that David's truck was gone. I found the ham in the oven, the beans on the stove and the corn bread on the counter. Delightful! It was lukewarm at best, but good food and I was hungry. So I fixed myself a plate and sat down to eat. I had been so looking forward to this.

I took my time eating, but no David. More time went by. Still no David. About half an hour later, David finally arrived, carrying a grocery bag bulging with an obvious half gallon of ice cream. Also in the bag? Ham. David said that he had gone out to get the ham. He said that he had looked at the beans and he had looked at the cornbread that he had made and decided that what they really needed was a ham to go with them!

I told him that was interesting because I had already eaten some ham for dinner.

"Where did you get it?" he asks.

"I got it in the oven," I reply.

"In this oven?" he asks.

"Yes."

"Well, where in the oven?" He opens the door to the oven. "It must have been in the way back."

"No," I say, "it was sitting right there on the oven shelf."

"Did I put it there?"

"Yes, you put it there."

"Oh, I must have forgotten."

So, now we have more ham to eat and the good intentions and good effort David put out to make dinner in the first place is lost. It was both funny and sad.

So, we have lots of ham, lots of sausages, lots of ketchup bottles, lots of Little Debbie Snack Cakes, lots of soda and lots of margarine. The food themes continue as David makes his daily pilgrimages to the store. I wonder if the store clerks wonder why he buys the same things over and over. Why am I so critical? I should count myself lucky that we are not starving and my shopping list is at least reduced by not having to purchase these items.

✦ ✦ ✦ ✦ ✦ ✦

I did go to that Alzheimer's presentation. It was actually very good. The social worker who presented it, as I learned later, heads up the local Alzheimer's agency. She seemed particularly interested in David's early onset and said that she would like to have us both join a group of similar people on the Cape. The prevalence of Alzheimer's on Cape Cod is high. Of course, the population here is older, but she said that even early onset numbers seem to be higher here.

We saw the movie *Complaints of a Dutiful Daughter*. It was much different in some ways and much the same in other ways. This woman's mother had Alzheimer's Disease, and like David, she sounded quite sane. She could explain away anything and make almost anything make sense—at least to her. David is like that. He plays educator. It could be full of fluff, but he makes it sound serious and real and worth your time to listen, when, in fact, it is a total waste of time and a waste of human thought. The great lesson for the daughter, delivered quite eloquently, was that her mother's quality of life was okay, acceptable and even enjoyable when judged by her mother, but demeaning, boring and empty when judged by the daughter.

That was meaningful to me. I do judge David by my own idea of what is appropriate. He is otherwise perfectly happy in many ways. I am the unhappy one. I am the one who has lost out on so much and cannot seem to find peace with anything anymore.

✦ ✦ ✦ ✦ ✦ ✦

I have decided to list my resentments. I have *so* many resentments.

I resent that David does not work over the winter. That he does not see any lack of ethics in accepting his unemployment check

74

and sitting on his ass for five months out of the year. What this has to do with his illness, I don't know, but I list it anyway because it bothers me.

I resent that David sleeps like he is on holiday each and every day. I resent that he does not get up in the mornings with me (if for nothing other than to not appear to look so lazy and to at least look somewhat supportive of my having to get up). No, instead he grabs my pillow as soon as my head leaves it, then rolls himself into the quilt and turns over.

I resent that David has bad breath from the Aricept that he takes or maybe it's the antidepressant he takes. He never used to have bad breath.

I resent that David eats truckloads of Toaster Strudels and Little Debbies. I resent that he drinks gallons of coffee. I resent that he is otherwise never hungry and that the concept of meals is so totally foreign to him most of the time.

I resent that David is no longer the man who used to fix things, make things, solve problems or do heavy lifting. Two years ago, he pulled out a ceiling to fix a plumbing leak that never existed in the first place. The ceiling is still missing. He hung a door that did not fit. He never took it down. It still hangs mismatched in the doorway that now lacks all the trim work that used to make it look somewhat good and somewhat normal.

The workshop still has a work table created by laying an extremely heavy door on top of stacks of plastic milk crates. It was supposed to be temporary, but temporary has turned into permanent. David says that he likes it just fine the way it is. Not that long ago, it would have been built with heavy two-by-fours and extra buttressed supports. Not only that, but the two-by-fours would likely be sanded smooth and stained or painted. No matter. No one can circumnavigate the work bench anyway because it is so full of boxes of junk that David can no longer organize or put away. It is a useless workshop. I *so* resent the useless wonderful workshop that we spent so much money to build!

I resent that David does the dishes and washes the kitchen floor to excess. That is what is most important to him. He mixes up the dishes in the cupboard. He folds the clothes into neat tight little piles. I want him to sand the floor and patch the roof, even though I know that he will never do those things again.

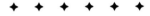

Two days ago, we got 12 inches of snow. David was meticulously cleaning off my car after I had already removed the heaviest snow. I told him that I needed him to help shovel the driveway so I could get to work the next morning.

"Do you have to manage everything?" he exclaimed angrily. "What possible difference does it make that I clean off the car first?"

After watching him a while more, I slunk off into the house. Of course, what difference does it make? None. Only at 5:45 the next morning, I went out to let the dogs out and to get the newspaper. There was the driveway waiting for me to shovel with its lovely 12 inches of snow. *Yes, you got it right, David.*

I do have to manage everything, and yes, it does make a difference. Don't you get it? You have the muscles! I needed you to shovel the driveway, not clean off my car. I could have cleaned off my car. So you cleaned off my car, but you forgot the driveway.

I guess that's something else I resent. David looks physically healthy. Here is someone who abused alcohol for many years and smoked two packs a day for over 30 years. He looks terrific! Alzheimer's does nothing to make him look sick at all. He will live to 100! I will die of stress and fatigue taking care of him.

Maybe I will just die of all my resentments. If not, I'll certainly never get past purgatory for being so bad or thinking such bad thoughts.

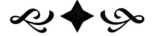

Every once in a while, David has an off day that hits those extreme alarm bells in my heart. I can actually feel my heart dancing off into tight corners with little twinges of pain that preach to me that I must understand that this is serious business. That there are consequences and an impact from this disease, and we cannot just go on living our lives as normal. It's not that some serious incident occurs. Instead, it is clear that David has retreated into his own world. He is so very distant from me at times.

I imagine sometimes that I will come home from work to find that David never got up. He died in his sleep. What would cause him to die? Well, since this is real, those brain cell connectors that are now glutenized may at some point glutenize some very vital communication in his brain. Like brain to lung—"Breathe in," lung to brain—"Okay, I did," brain to lung—"Now breathe out," lung to brain—"Okay, I did,"…and so on.

He wouldn't have to miss too many of those communications to do some irreversible damage.

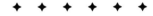

It's March and, very soon, David will go back to work. We don't know when. David will not call his boss to find out. Instead, he will sit around waiting for the call. Since he doesn't have much to do while he's waiting, I come up with a list of things that he can do before he returns to work. One thing on the list is to rent a carpet cleaner and clean all the rugs in the house. There really aren't that many and our house is not that big. It should be doable.

So, David musters up some energy and seems quite into it. He rents the machine and buys a small bottle of rug shampoo. I notice that he is bent over reading the instructions on the machine for a very long time. Finally, he seems satisfied that he needs to vacuum first, so he takes our big vacuum upstairs. Then he comes back and grabs the little vacuum and takes that upstairs as well. It's really just a bare floor quick sweeper. He uses the big vacuum in one room then uses the little vacuum in the other room. When he realizes that the little vacuum is not very effective on the rug upstairs, he comes back downstairs to get the kitchen floor scrubber. That's a new little machine we have had since Christmas. It does vacuum, but it's not meant for rugs. We got it to scrub (as in wash) the tile floor in the kitchen. I'm not sure why we have so many cleaning tools in the first place, but we do. Probably just like everyone else, we were sucked in by a TV ad and then waited for the item to show up at our local department store on sale.

I ask David why he wants to take the floor scrubber upstairs. He says that he needs to vacuum.

"Why don't you use the big vacuum you left in the other room upstairs?" I ask.

"What?" he replies, obviously annoyed.

I try again. "Why don't you use the big vacuum you left in the other room upstairs?"

"I didn't know there was a big vacuum in the other room."

"But you vacuumed the rug in there." Now I'm annoyed.

"I did?"

"Yes, you did."

"Oh, okay."

Ten minutes later, David comes downstairs and says that he should go out to get "that sprinkle stuff that you put on the rugs to make them smell good".

"Why would you do that when you are going to shampoo the rugs?" I ask.

"I am?" he replies.

"Yes."

"How would I do that?" he asks.

"With the carpet cleaner that you rented." I reply very matter-of-factly. I am now his teacher, his repeater, his matter-of-facter. Why am I pushing back like this?

"I did?" he responds. I could swear I've heard this before. We are going around in circles.

I try again. "Yes, you did. You just brought it home today. That is why you are vacuuming the rugs—to get ready to shampoo the rugs."

"Oh, okay."

This nearly exact conversation is actually repeated three times over the course of the night and I am exhausted by it.

I wonder why I'm contented to let him take on such a big job by himself but then I'm not very supportive when he runs into problems. Secretly, I think I am just hopeful that he will figure things out and I won't have to get involved. But then, having to stop and give him directions makes it seem just not worth it after all. I get disrupted in whatever I am trying to get done and then, it's like talking to a wall. I just can't get through. Or maybe I do get through, but it's later according to David's timeline, like tomorrow morning when I'm back at work. By tomorrow morning, somehow, magically, some of the carpets will be clean. I can only hope.

✦　✦　✦　✦　✦　✦

Much later that night, David becomes very argumentative. He was using our best china to feed the cat wet canned fish food. I asked him why he didn't use one of the animal bowls.

"What animal bowls?" he asks.

"The blue bowls," I reply.

"The blue bowls are animal bowls? No one ever told me that."

"Well, they are." I'm getting good at this matter-of-facting.

"Since when?" he argues.

"Hmmm. For ten years or so. For ten years we have used the blue plastic bowls to feed the animals. We don't use those bowls. The animals use those bowls." Again, I'm so good with the facts.

"Then why are they in the cabinet?" He just wants to make trouble.

"Because you put them there." Do I have to spell it out for him?

"If they are animal bowls, why are they in the cabinet?" Another argument.

"Well, I never wanted them in there, but you kept putting them in there, so I gave up." I shoot my reply back with poison darts attached.

Then gruffly, he is looking for scissors and complaining that there are never any scissors in the house when he needs them. Why is that? I explain that they are not here in the kitchen and I have not yet found the most recent place where he has rounded them all up to live.

"What?"

"Yes, you gather together things like pens and scissors and then you put them all together in one place. I just haven't found out yet where you have stored all the scissors." Another fact.

"Well, that's because they will fall over," David explains. "If you put the scissors into a jar like that, they will fall over and the scissors will fall out onto the floor. That's why I never put the scissors in those jars over there. I won't do it because it's dangerous."

He is becoming quite adept at rationalizing in a most interesting but crazy way.

✦ ✦ ✦ ✦ ✦ ✦

Later, I ask David if he would like to see the pictures from Kristin's bridal shower.

"Yes."

He is squinting at one photograph.

"Oh, that looks nice. Where was this? Why is it all decorated?"

"It's at the restaurant and it's decorated for Kristin's bridal shower."

He squints at another picture. "Is that my daughter?"

My heart sinks. "Yes," I reply.

"Oh, doesn't she look nice."

"Yes."

✦ ✦ ✦ ✦ ✦ ✦

Tonight, David came home from the store with two bags of groceries. He opened the cookbook to a page with a recipe that he wanted to cook. He said, "Well, if you want to help me cook this, I could use the help."

This was a nice change from fighting with each other. I started to work with him, putting on some rice to cook. I cleaned the fish, and then cut the fish into cubes.

David is starting to get very agitated. I ask if he would like me to chop the garlic or make the chicken broth? His brow is furrowed.

"What's wrong?" I ask.

"Well, that's why I like to get everything ready before I start," he says.

"What do you mean?"

"Well, like the garlic. I chop it up before I start."

"Yes, well, that is what I was going to help you with. What's the problem?"

"The problem is you starting things. I need to have everything ready at the same time."

"Well, I started the rice, because it takes 25 minutes to cook. I thought that the fish and asparagus would take less time than that, so it would be a good idea to get the rice started first. Even if the rice is ready ahead of time, it will sit in the covered pan and stay hot for up to 20 minutes, so it is no problem if it's cooked ahead of time." I offered my reasons in a dispassionate manner; but in truth, I knew that this endeavor at cooking together in a friendly, harmoniously married manner was not going to work.

David is moving things around on the counter with his brow furrowed.

I shut off the rice and leave the room.

Half an hour later, David comes in and says that dinner is ready and he is sorry that he was in a bad mood. He was just feeling like things were getting out of control.

I realized after dinner that the reason the fish tasted so bland was that David never did chop the garlic and he never did fix the broth that was supposed to be part of the recipe he wanted to cook. He just left those items out.

Oh well. Another night in our lives confused, wasted with fighting or just simply being disagreeable with each other. Neither of us can seem to put the brakes on. Why is that?

I am having a lot of trouble thinking about how I can be less clear and less logical so as not to arouse David's anger. We oppose each other all the time now. He with his cob-webbed brain and me with my thinking brain. He absolutely hates that my brain still works and his does not. He gets angry when I make sense. I get angry when he doesn't make sense.

While I was reading through this tonight, David has come into the room at least four times so far. He is playing with the cat. I think he is curious about what I am typing. I think he knows what I'm typing. I have password-protected this file, but it wouldn't take much for him to figure out my password. He is still so smart and yet so foggy. It is such a dichotomy and so very hard to live with.

Do I know why I'm writing this? It's something about needing to write it all down because I just don't know what's ahead. Maybe I think in some odd way that if I have a record of the past, somehow I will be able to understand the future.

At some point, I will be able to understand this, and then maybe I won't be so scared all the time.

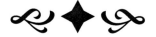

Today, David has an appointment with his neurologist. He not only remembered to go with only three paper reminders hung around the kitchen, he was there on time and was having a good old time with the doctor by the time I got there to join him. The no-bedside-manner-gloom-and-doom doctor was laughing it up with David over something funny. Maybe I shouldn't be going to these appointments?

The doctor ran David through the same gamut of tests. He could not spell the word "WORLD" backwards or remember the three words he was asked to remember. He got the day of the week right this time, but the date wrong, or vice versa. Again, I sat there trying not to laugh out loud. It seemed so much the same to me. And that was exactly the way it turned out. So many more months down the road on Aricept and he seems to be holding his own. This is very good news. He has not gotten any worse!

In fact, when David had this appointment, about three weeks ago now, he was really into his spry time of year. All perked up getting ready to get back to work. It's like he comes out of a deep sleep. For a while at least, he was so much more responsive and alert.

But that was temporary. Now we are back into really, really bad moods and lots of blaming and complaining. He gets mad at me. I get mad at him. Lisa gets mad at me for getting mad at him. I get mad at Lisa for getting mad at me. It's a damn vicious cycle! She doesn't see any of the day-to-day, except when she is visiting here from Boston. I do not know how to stop reacting and sometimes, I don't even know how or why we get into verbal challenges.

I reach for a bowl. A glass vase crashes to the floor in the kitchen.

"Damn. Someone put a glass vase inside this bowl," I exclaim.

David says, "What?"

"Someone put a glass vase inside this bowl where you can't see it up on the top shelf. I went to take down the bowl and out came the glass vase. There was no way I could have seen it. How could I have seen it?"

David's response is: "It's no wonder. It's all trash. This whole thing is shoddy. It's a shoddy mess. Look. Look at this. Should this be up there?" David takes a glass quart jar down from the shelf.

"Yes. Why not?" I'm a little hesitant in my reply. I don't see where he is going with this.

"Well, because it's glass. Gah-lass! So, it shouldn't be up there either, right?"

"I can see that it's glass. I can see it on the shelf. I would know to be careful of it. The glass vase that broke was hidden *inside* the bowl." I keep trying to explain things, but he is not getting it.

"So none of this should be up here, right? It's a mess. It's all going to fall down. But, no. You keep putting things up there. You don't want to fix it. Where else should it have gone? There's no room for anything else. This whole shelf is going to fall down."

"Stop it, David."

"What's wrong? You think you can put things anywhere you want? When there's no room? There's no room to put anything in this house."

"Stop it, David." I demand again. I do not want to hear this.

"Why? Okay, fine. You won't listen. It's no wonder this place is such a mess. You put all this stuff around."

With that, he walks out of the kitchen. I go get the vacuum to vacuum up the broken glass. Maybe he put the glass vase inside the bowl. Maybe he didn't. I have to learn not to make any remarks about anything or it will turn into warfare.

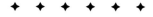

I realize that the house that I used to love and now worry about constantly has been doomed to David's negativity. It can never be a nice place again. Everything is falling down or rotting or collapsing or leaking. Whether it really is or not, that is how he sees it, and I think I have totally adopted that perspective. Now, I'm very unhappy in this house.

Mostly, this is a dangerous house for David. Too dangerous. He has already made too many mistakes trying to fix things he no longer understands. There are so many things awaiting repair. The shop is full of dangerous tools. Maybe the only answer is to move away from it all and start clean, in a much safer environment for David. I wonder, *If we sell this house and move to a newer house, will that house suffer the same fate? And if so, how long will it take? Could we squeeze a few good years out of it?*

✦　✦　✦　✦　✦　✦

Kristin was married two days ago in a beautiful ceremony.

David walked her down the aisle, but when he got to the end of it, he didn't know what to do. He didn't even kiss her or hug her. He kind of moved a little back and a little off to the side. I tugged at the end of his jacket and finally got his attention to move him to a chair. Later, when pictures were taken, David was the ultimate goofball. He had a silly grin on his face for most of the pictures. He would send up an arm or leg in the middle of a photo setting. Twice, I saw the photographer actually pull him by the sleeve out of the photo shoot. It was fine though, because David never realized what was happening. He had a good time at the wedding. To me, it was oddly like a shell of him was there and he really wasn't there. No one else noticed. Many people complimented him and told me how well he looked.

I interpreted these communications as, *What are you, crazy? He doesn't look sick!*

90

So I am home today, putting away all the collected wedding things like decorations and ribbons and packaging up the tuxedos to take back. David did not participate in a single wedding preparation, except to help me pre-sample the wedding cake. If there had been no wedding, he would not have noticed.

I go to put the dishes away in the cupboard. They are dirty. The dishes that David prides himself on washing in near boiling water are just not clean. He has started to use a stiff brush instead of a sponge. Once he locks onto something that he thinks is a good idea, he will not let go of it. So, now I will have to add to my chores the task of re-washing the dishes after he goes to bed. I will just have to be careful not to make any remarks about them!

I can see, reading all this over, that David is into a better stage now that he has been on Aricept for almost a year. It is also springtime, which is historically David's best time of the year and his least likely time to be depressed. Also, he is stimulated by the fact that Brandon is now staying with us and that helps as well. Brandon is our nephew from Texas whom we raised for many years. He comes back home to roost periodically. He is just beginning to understand that David really does have an illness and he will do things like leave the stove on or forget to eat or forget where he put things or get easily stressed from too much stimulation—like the TV blasting or two people talking at the same time.

Brandon and David have a good relationship, laughing and kidding with each other. I keep telling Brandon to be cautious because it may happen out of the blue that, very occasionally, David may do a really odd thing like forget what turn to take off Route 6A.

Once again, I feel like the streak of doom having to emphasize to other people that this is an illness and it's both routinely and unexpectedly difficult.

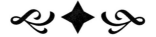

Up until July, David was doing well. Once he started back to work, he became a different person. He has not been as depressed or angry. He has been more alert and more focused. We are so lucky that his job is relatively safe. He takes a circuitous route from his dock, traveling through a connection of small bays on mostly calm waters and back to his dock, several times a day.

It's August now, though, and I can see that he does get quite physically tired. When he gets to the end of his five-day work week, he literally needs to go right to bed. He is that tired. But now, I am seeing other changes that have me very worried. We are back to "My God, this is a real disease and it is so unpredictable!" David appears to have fallen off some ledge. He is now in a fog more often.

I should note, as well, that David has now passed his milestone one-year anniversary on Aricept. Kris learned that there are statistics that show that Aricept has a clear indication of a good effect, peaking at one year and then falling again. As Kris put it, it is a temporary help at best, because David will get worse. The Aricept delays the inevitable, but the inevitable still happens. She is quite sad and shocked to finally grasp the idea that Alzheimer's is, in fact, a terminal illness. Odd to think of it that way. Don't we all have a terminal illness that may just be lying dormant right now? You just can't look at David and think that he may die from this. If anything, David is more handsome than ever with his summer tan. He is more active and has shed some of his winter ice-cream weight.

David is reminiscing more, thinking about good times we have had, particular places we have been, the Cape of yesterday that was so idyllic and less populated than it is now. He has gathered pictures together and displays them on his night table or in his jewelry box. He is quieter. There is no mistaking that he knows what is happening, and it is as though all the hard edges and the anger and the fight have all but disappeared. He is quieter, maybe more accepting. I don't necessarily take this as a good sign.

He continues to scrub the dishes with a hard brush, as he is convinced that sponges (and wooden cutting boards) are potentially toxic with bacteria. He's not wrong about the potential bacteria, but the hard brush just doesn't get the dishes clean and he can't be convinced that it might not be the best way to clean the dishes in the absence of a dishwasher.

More and more, David needs to see and focus on what I say. That is, he has to be looking at me. I have to be in his face talking directly to him so that he can absorb the words better. If I am turned to the side, he hears garble and asks me what I said. Sometimes, he cannot remember a simple word or phrase. He might say, "You know that holiday with the fireworks?" because he cannot remember the Fourth of July. He calls Stop & Shop the place where you go to buy food.

He is a coffee lover, but twice last week he left for work without pouring himself even one cup of coffee. He walked out on a full pot without a cup and without a thermos. I feel so sorry for him when things like that happen. What if he is out there on the water and suddenly realizes that his coffee is missing?

I still haven't figured out dinner time. I watch him turn in circles looking for something to latch onto that he is familiar with. It is most often the sink and washing any dishes that are in the sink. Sometimes, he will help me set the table, but not often. Then, when the food is ready, he does everything but sit down to eat. He looks for things...soda, paper towels, a serving spoon, or salt and pepper. I am a slow eater, but I am half done by the time he sits down. I have started to serve him on his plate. Maybe it is the idea of having to decide what to take, how much to take and how it should sit on his plate that disturbs him. I am not sure. He doesn't seem to mind me setting up his plate for him.

✦ ✦ ✦ ✦ ✦ ✦

We are at a turning point about to embark on a new phase of our lives in so many ways. The house has been on the market since July and now we have an offer. I was afraid that David would be quite upset about having to move, but he is truly delighted and excited by the prospect. Since security is everything now, I put in an offer on a new house before selling the old one and got a bridge loan to cover the expense until our house sells. It is such a scary prospect to be looking at an enormous monthly payment until this house sells, but it had to be this way. It's the only way to maintain a secure environment for David. So far, it seems like it was the right decision. David loves our new house and he is really looking forward to moving.

The new house has two bedrooms, a single-car garage, a full basement, a small family room and a beautiful Grandma-style screened-in porch with an exceptionally private back yard and an outside shower. It is everything we need and nothing we don't need. This house will cut down on the lawn mowing and on the maintenance nightmares that we have faced in a very old house. It immediately solves the problem of having a workshop full of saws and other dangerous equipment that David should not operate. All that will be replaced by a small basement workshop with the dangerous things mysteriously lost in the move. Best of all, the neighborhood road forms a large loop, which will be excellent for walking the dogs. That should help David to feel much more at ease, walking without any cars whizzing by, trying to hit him.

The move is less about where we are going and much more about cleaning up and clearing out. We are downsizing all of our accumulated stuff and David is pitching right in. Organizing things is very important to him so he is following my lead that we will keep 20 percent, put 20 percent in a yard sale and throw out 60 percent. We don't need five snow shovels and I guarantee that I will never use six socket sets with 150 pieces that no longer fit in the boxes. So much of this was inherited from my father, who kept everything and lived a very long life. We simply adopted all of it and never cleaned it up.

We look forward to the prospect of our own new little house together. It is very comforting to David. He clings to me a lot now for comfort, needing more hugs recently, holding on to me at night, welcoming me home. It's very clear that the world is starting to become a scary place for him.

✦ ✦ ✦ ✦ ✦ ✦

A few weeks ago, David started having bad dreams. Really scary nightmare dreams that he could not get out of his head when he woke up in the morning. At first, he wouldn't talk about them—but said they were about things affecting us, his family. A few nights ago, it was work. It's September now, and he is nearing the end of the boating season. He thought he had made a mess of his end-of-year report and lost or garbled his data. He got up to find that it wasn't true, but he was so troubled that he could not go to work.

This was unthinkable that David would not be able to go to work. He kept saying that he had "anxiety" and he could not make the feeling go away. So he stayed home and I called his doctor. His doctor recommended that David go to ½ a dose of Aricept. We started that yesterday, so we will see if that makes a difference. We'll see his doctor again in a couple of weeks.

Last night, I came home and opened the refrigerator door to take out the small steak I had moved from the freezer that morning, expecting to cook it for dinner. Instead, there was hamburger in the refrigerator. David said that he had been to the store and wasn't it good that he had bought the ground sirloin that was on the list?

I told him there was no ground sirloin on the list. I asked him if he had seen the steak that was defrosting in the refrigerator. He said, "What steak? I didn't see any steak. Are you sure you put it in the refrigerator?"

"Yes, I'm positive," I said.

David repeated my search of the refrigerator and then searched the freezer. I searched the freezer.

No steak. I asked, "Did you throw it away?"

"No. Well, it was probably me. I was probably the one who fucked up. I'm so sick of this."

This makes me sad. I'm sad when David thinks of things in this way. I actually prefer it when he fights me or challenges what I say because that means that he is fighting the illness too.

So, maybe he threw it away or set it down in a cabinet, and we will smell it well before we find it, or maybe it will just turn up.

And it did turn up. I made the hamburgers for dinner and when I went to heat up a cup of coffee in the microwave, there was the steak! David had put it in there to defrost about two hours ago. He just didn't remember.

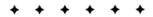

I ask David more questions about troubles he may be having at work. He says the trouble is that people keep moving their boats so he doesn't always know where to find them. He is having trouble keeping up with the radio reports that give him the name of the boat to pump out and the location. He comes home with this information written in ink across his hands. What would be better? *Could people call in their requests to the main office and then he could pick up the written requests from the office? Yes, that would work better. Do you want me to talk to your boss about it? Yes, would you?*

If I talk to David's boss, that may be the end of David's job, although David says that he has explained to people at work that he has memory problems, and he does get a fair amount of help at times, particularly from the ladies in the office. Still, his coworkers may not think it's a good idea for someone with Alzheimer's to be out on a boat. I would agree, except that this job is David's lifeline. Without it, he will not last very long. I just know it. He will decline so fast. So, I have to figure out how to accomplish this and save David's job at the same time or find him an easier job and do the negotiating for him.

In mid-September, I write this letter to David's doctor, but end up not giving it to him. I am so undecided about what I should do for David. I need to write it all down to think it through myself, to analyze the situation.

Dear Doctor:

David has become very anxious and paranoid to the extent that it overwhelms him and he cannot be relieved from the severe anxiety that he feels. He sleeps fitfully and he has repeated bad dreams. When he gets up in the morning, he is gritting his teeth and totally unable to relax to any degree.

Overall, David was doing remarkably well up through June. He has perceptibly declined since then with even shorter memory and great anxiety over the upcoming end of his seasonal work for the town as an assistant harbormaster. It is particularly the report that will be due in about five weeks that has him feeling that he cannot cope and that he will be fired. This has never caused him a problem before. David no longer reads much and he does no writing at all except for grocery lists. He has started to fish for words—like the post office may be "that place where you drop off letters."

David does have most of the information he needs to write this report for work, but he truly believes that he has made a complete mess of it, that he is failing to do his job, that his boss will be mad and that the town will lose funds. I reassure him constantly, but it does no good. I have reviewed his paperwork and I have had another person review it. Although he is missing some data, it is not a complete mess at all. We will help him do the report.

On your recommendation, we cut his dose of Aricept in half, but I see no difference and David has asked to be put back on the full dose. He is unable to tell me what he is feeling other than the above extreme anxiety. I ask him how he is feeling and he says, "I forget."

What I also see is that he has changed recently and that he is very scared, clinging, insecure and worried about dying.

What I would ask is the following:
> *Perhaps some anti-anxiety medication to give him some immediate relief.*
> *A note for David to bring to work that will allow him to take sick leave for the rest of this season (which will end approximately mid-Oct). He has the sick leave to take. He is asking me if he can stay home—absolutely uncharacteristic!*

I would like his job to understand that he may be going through a temporary unstable phase, and he needs the time to get his medications adjusted. I do not want them to assume that he can no longer work.

We have a complicated process to go through to allow David to apply for total disability under the town retirement system. David first has to buy back some time from prior military employment and then go through the four-month process to be declared totally disabled. We will likely need medical documentation from you supporting his disability.

I have never seen David in such an alarming state of inability to cope. The last thing I would want to see is for David to have to end his employment because that is what keeps him going and he loves his job. Once he is no longer working, he will decline even more rapidly. We are both well aware of this fact, so this is a very difficult situation.

He currently only takes the Aricept, an aspirin, a multivitamin, and Saw Palmetto. Is it possible that this extreme anxiety could be a temporary situation that may improve with some other medication?

Thanks for your attention to this. David has an appointment with you at the end of September. Should we try to move that up?

Sincerely,

Instead of giving this to his doctor, I used it for talking points. Staying home from work was so unlike David. He could not even dial the phone to call his boss to tell him he needed a day off. I had to call in for him. The doctor started David on Paxil to help reduce his anxiety. Five days later, David says he is feeling better, less worried and more focused. He returns to work.

✦ ✦ ✦ ✦ ✦ ✦

Reporting for duty is not something you mess with. That's the military in David. He will go to work with a temperature of 104 degrees if that is where he is supposed to be. You don't let your boss down. You don't let your buddies down. You don't show weakness. You show resolve. It's about honor and dedication. It was difficult to talk David into believing that it was actually okay for him to take a day off once in a while. A sick day, a rest day. A few weeks later, David did take another sick day. He seemed so relieved not to have to go to work. Again, uncharacteristic, but so necessary.

I didn't want him to be alone. So, later in the day, I took him with me to babysit our grandson. He appeared to me to be comforted and able to function pretty well while with me. I am beginning to understand that he is developing a dependency on my presence to maintain his well-being. There were a few times that he was short-tempered when the jabber-jabber of a seven-year-old was more than he could take; but on the whole, he seemed to enjoy the day with us and function mostly in a focused manner.

I can't force him to quit his job, but I need to bring it up with him more often. Maybe then, it will ultimately become his own decision that he should no longer try to work. It will be a major adjustment for us financially, but there is no choice. I have the certain knowledge that it will happen, so it almost doesn't matter to me exactly when.

Year Three

Thinking of David not being able to work was just so foreign. He had always worked. When we met, he was in the Navy working as an enlisted electronics technician. After 10 years in the Navy, we left Hawaii, and David left the Navy to explore other career options. It seemed like an opportune time to try something new. We had both finished our undergraduate degrees while attending evening classes at one of the Army bases in Hawaii. David had then gone on to complete a special weekend extension program that earned him a Master's Degree in Education from Pepperdine University. By then, he had migrated out of electronics work. He was editor of the base newspaper and he ran race relations education seminars for enlisted staff and officers.

One of the career options he had in his back pocket was attending Officer Candidate School for the Coast Guard. We had met a wonderful Coast Guard family and David was really drawn to the mission and the chance to work closer to our eventual home on the East Coast. So he applied, not really thinking that he would get in. To his great surprise, he was selected from an impossibly large pool of candidates. That made it seem even more special, so off David went to Norfolk, Virginia, while I returned to my parents' home outside of Boston with two small children in tow to wait out the four months that David was in school.

For the next decade, David worked as a training officer for the Coast Guard headquarters in Washington, D.C., and then as a training officer for the First Coast Guard district in Boston. Toward the end of his tour in Boston, we were finally able to return to Cape Cod, where we had always planned to live.

After retiring from the Coast Guard, there were quite a few years in between when David could not attach himself to any job with much enthusiasm, so the jobs didn't last very long. He sold marine electronics, office products, and even tried to sell cars. For a few years, he worked as a manager for Radio Shack. It was a good job for him with his technical background, strong computer knowledge and his extraordinary social skills. But as he entered his mid-40s, some problems developed. I was totally unaware of the significance at the time. It was only years later that I made the connection.

David worked 11-hour days for Radio Shack, six days a week. I wasn't very tolerant of this work schedule, but he said that was what it took to keep his store running. He had to keep things ship-shape in true military fashion, so how could I argue? Plus, he was a hard worker and he was determined to do things right. Eventually, I realized that managing his store's inventory was proving to be difficult. There would be stacks of boxes in the back room, some going out for repair, some coming in for restocking. David was obviously stressed when inventory counts had to be taken. I would join his staff for the overnight counts. He would laugh and joke his way through these nights, while I seemed to be doing more and more to organize his work and keep it moving along. David was, in fact, shoring up his coping skills, just managing to get by to get the work done. He was already losing his organizational skills that had always been so strong, only neither of us knew that this was happening at the time. It was just taking more and more time to do what he used to be able to do in a snap.

When the assistant harbormaster job came along, it was a godsend. It was much more of what David really needed, being outside on the water and talking with people. It was much less of the stressors of managing inventory and paperwork. He excelled in marine safety; he knew the regulations and the electronics, and he was an exceptional boat operator. He also carried with him a long career of honor and discipline that made every task one that he took on with pride. He was in uniform again and he felt very much at home.

So, thinking about David having to eventually leave this job which had been a source of comfort and strength for him was both sad and upsetting.

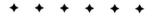

David did complete his season of work for the town, and he completed his report just fine. In the end, he was quite proud of his accomplishments and admitted that he had been going through a temporary period of anxiety that had him unnecessarily worried.

During his layoff season, we were working so hard together on preparing for our move that David didn't have time to be morose or sullen. With the help of our son-in-law Dennis, we did quite a lot of upgrading to the house before we moved in. Dennis and David got along great, always laughing and joking with each other. I love that Dennis never once showed any impatience with David. David held wood pieces for Dennis while he cut and framed a new closet and put up crown molding. David eagerly took on the tasks of cleaning up and making runs to Dunkin' Donuts for coffee and hot chocolate.

I worried about David on the road, but Dennis thought he was still doing fine in that regard. It would be a hard thing to take away his truck. David was so proud of his truck. In addition to being an excellent boat operator, David was also an excellent driver. Wherever we went, David always did the driving. I had to agree with Dennis that, although I had seen some problems, it was not the time to tackle this issue with David. After all, if he couldn't drive, he couldn't work.

Just after the new year, David started a new medication called Namendia. It's supposed to be like a booster to the Aricept, giving him more time with improved symptoms. I don't like that he has definitely added a streak of meanness on this medication. He acts like I am harassing him when I just ask a question. He wants to know what does it matter? Why does he have to explain what he does or why he does it? He sits down to dinner and feeds himself and never tells me that dinner is ready. When I ask him why he does not tell me that dinner is ready, he scowls at me. "Why should I have to tell you dinner is ready?" Tonight, he shut off all the lights on me and went to bed. He did the same thing two nights ago.

Tonight, he said he would set the table for dinner but didn't do it. When I asked him about it, he said, "Well, maybe I didn't get to it, did you think of that?" in a nasty tone of voice. He opened the cabinet and pulled down two plates for us for dinner, a small plate and a dinner plate and put them on the counter. I asked why he was using a small plate. He said, "What does it matter?" I explained that we use dinner-sized plates at dinner. He made a remark about my rules and having to live by all my rules. He said all the plates we have are junk anyway and there are no two matching plates. (There are several.)

When he eats lately, he literally shovels food in and he has a big crease in his brow. He does not talk to me or engage in any type of conversation. He seems to walk purposefully with a mean look. Even when Kris and Dennis and Devon are here, he seems to ignore them, focusing on his serious task, whatever it is. In our new house, we have a dishwasher, which he routinely fills and refills. Dishes are getting washed over and over again. He walks from one counter to the other, pours a glass of soda water, back to the den, back to the counter. It is not clear what the task is. By then, he has forgotten what it is, so it looks like purposeful wandering.

He seems to relish making a mess or making me upset, I am not sure which one. David has boots with big treads in the soles that pick up clogs of dirt. He walks purposely from outside to inside and then throughout the house. When I ask why he doesn't seem to care what he is doing, he says that is the way it is. His boots track dirt. So what? He has no other shoes. Of course he has other shoes! He is just being difficult.

This is someone I don't know and don't like. It's as though he is as disgusted as hell all the time and he is striking out against all of us. I particularly feel sorry for our grandson, Devon. We used to all be so happy together playing ball in the front yard, playing board games on the table in the den. Now, David freely expresses his annoyance with Devon. When Devon comes over, David retreats to our bedroom. It's not as though Devon doesn't notice that his grandfather doesn't like him anymore. His own behavior is becoming challenging and disrespectful. Yet, is it Devon's fault? He's the child. I can't blame him.

Routinely now, David can no longer do a large grocery shopping like he used to like to do. He cannot concentrate on a long list, so he just stops at some point. Only about half of what he buys now matches the list that he went in with. He is still buying the same things over and over again. If he bought chicken yesterday, he will buy chicken today. He lives on junk food—adding donuts and varieties of Chex Mix to his diet of Little Debbies and ice cream. Last week he surprised himself with how much ice cream he had bought. He filled the freezer. I found out later that he gave some of it away to Kristin. So he is aware, even though he is not talking about it. He is aware that something is wrong.

Dennis took David to the Fishing Expo in Boston. It was great for me because it gave me a break, a chance to be alone. Dennis mentioned when they came home that David had made an inappropriate remark to a vendor they had been talking to. David said, "Goodbye, ugly," when they were leaving. Of course, the vendor had a bit of a perplexed look in response to this out-of-the-blue remark. I told Dennis that it is just a variation of a theme with David. When he cannot remember someone's name, he will call them something else that he makes up and sometimes it's derogatory. My dog is "Squirt." His friend from the Navy is "Buggerbrain." Most of the time, he is laughing and so we laugh right along with him. This was different, though, because it was out in public. That made it different and significant.

✦ ✦ ✦ ✦ ✦ ✦

We are settled in to our new house and neighborhood and very happy. David is much more comfortable walking the dog around our closed neighborhood loop. There is no way to get lost and there are very few cars driving past.

I so clearly remember trying to keep up with David's pace as we walked together only a year ago. For so many years, we had walked at different times of the day, and I always thought I was a fast walker until I joined David on his walks in the evenings last year. I could barely keep up with him. His stride just seemed so smooth and quick that I would be panting trying to keep up.

Now I easily outpace him around our new neighborhood. *When did that happen? When did he slow down so much?* I keep asking him if he is tired. He says no and looks at me quizzically. I have tried to match my stride with his, stride for stride. I can't quite figure out what he is doing differently, but there is absolutely no doubt that his pace has significantly slowed down.

✦ ✦ ✦ ✦ ✦ ✦

David saw a new primary care doctor today. The new doctor came highly recommended by Kristin, who has worked with him and watched him with Alzheimer's patients at the nursing home where she works. When the doctor entered the room, David was telling me some story that I can't even remember now, but it was very unimportant. He never even looked up to greet the doctor, but kept on talking to me. I interrupted him and said, "David, this is the doctor." It was only then that he stopped talking and greeted the doctor. I thought he was otherwise pretty normal through the appointment, but on thinking back, I guess David was unable to answer some questions, so the doctor would look to me for the answers. We talked openly about David's Alzheimer's Disease and his current symptoms and medications. David gave the doctor complete freedom to talk with me and with Kristin about his condition.

Apparently, the doctor told Kris later that he was quite surprised at how advanced David was into this disease. He was particularly surprised, because he is in very good health otherwise. He figured that David is three years away from having to be in a nursing home. He also said that he is 100 percent disabled and that he should not be returning to work and he should not be driving. He ordered complete blood work and will do a physical at the end of April. We were a bit taken aback by his assessment as, so far, it has sort of been status quo. Most of the time, I feel it is me and me alone being wary about David's future and my own. It is me thinking that this illness is really more than it is. Other people don't see it. Well, somehow, the doctor saw it.

Again, that fleeting dose of reality.

✦ ✦ ✦ ✦ ✦ ✦

Kris called me at work and wanted to know what was I doing to prepare for this eventuality of having to put her dad into a nursing home in only three years? What had I done about this? Obviously, doing anything at work or from work would have been out of the question, and there are very long answers to such a question. The quick answer had to be, "I don't know." And in truth, I am lost. But I completely understood Kristin's stress-provoked foraging into the future. We can't just sit around and not prepare for this.

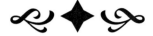

So far, I know a few things. I know that David cannot qualify for long-term-care insurance, so that's out. I also know that David does not qualify for Social Security Disability. Even though his doctor says he is 100 percent disabled and even though David has over 35 years of contributions to the Social Security system behind him, he is not eligible. Over the past nine years, he has worked for a municipality, and they do not contribute to the Social Security system. Without contributions during the years just preceding his disability, he cannot qualify. Who thought up this rule and why? It makes no sense. I don't understand how or why it exists, but it does exist. David is just not a candidate for Social Security Disability. How many doors does that close for him? Right now, I don't know.

So, I have been working on pulling together the information we will need for David to qualify for a small disability retirement from the state retirement system through the town where he has worked. There is something called "Ordinary Disability" that David can qualify for with 10 years of service. I have already put through the paperwork that will give him retirement credits for four years of military service. That will put him over the 10-year mark in the retirement system. It makes me wonder, of course, what do people do who have less than 10 years' municipal service? It's a black hole. I count our blessings that it seems that David should qualify for this disability income, but we will have to go through all the hoops to apply for it and to be approved.

I tell David what I'm doing, researching this option. He doesn't automatically connect it with not returning to work. I won't even go there anyhow, because I don't know how long this may take. I may have to get an attorney. We are just at the beginning of this process. Most of the time, David is very trusting when it comes to my handling of our personal affairs, bill paying, savings and such. He is trusting about this as well. Or, does he not understand what I'm talking about and so he can't argue? I just don't know.

I also looked up info on Veteran's medical benefits, but that will take me a while to understand. It seems to be a very cumbersome system with a lot to read through. A door has closed on some eligibility already, as there are too many veterans seeking care. David needs to "enroll." There is no automatic consideration for retired military people with 20 years' service to receive VA medical care, at least not for long-term-care benefits. I have sent away for the enrollment paperwork. At least I'll start with that.

✦ ✦ ✦ ✦ ✦ ✦

I'm playing doctor. It's March 3 and today I removed David's morning Namendia pills. So as of today, he is down to just an evening 10-milligram pill for the next four or five days and then I will pull that one as well. Actually, I had reported David's negativity, anger and aggressiveness to his doctor, and he felt that it was fine to take David off this medication. I was actually going to wait a bit more. David does seem more alert, but it is not a positive thing. He is trying to do things that are beyond his skill level and that stresses him out.

The other night, he was determined to cook a new dish that was not so complicated in itself, but it did have multiple ingredients and multiple steps. David had the ingredients, pans, bowls, measuring cups and spoons strewn from one end of the kitchen to the other. It's sad to see him try so hard only to be lost in his own confusion. Constantly he would have to check and recheck where he was and what he was supposed to do next. He did cook the dish, but the pasta was too undercooked for me to eat much of it. So, it's good that he is still trying to cook, I guess, but bad that it's too much for him.

David's negativity has increased. Last night was an example. When I came in the door from work, he raised his voice to a firm loud pitch—not yelling exactly, but a forceful tone. "Why is this on the counter? I don't get it. How did this get here? I know you are going to blame me for it. You always do. I did not do this. You can blame me for other things, but you cannot blame me for this." What he was pointing to was a plastic container with one pill for Annie's inflammatory bowel disease.

It has occurred to me that the dog's intestinal disease could possibly be in response to our constantly nagging at each other. She has developed this disease over time. While I understand that it is a true hardship for David to stay out of taking care of Annie, given that she is his dog, I have been adamant that he must let me handle the dog's medication doses. For the mid-day dose, I leave a container of food with the medication in the food and put that on the counter for David to give to the dog. That is the only thing he needs to do.

Well, David does give it to the dog, one piece of food at a time. He says this is how the dog likes it and wants it and this is how it should be. He feeds the ¾ cup of dry kibble to the dog, one piece at a time. When he gets to the pills, he makes sure the dog swallows the pills. I tell David that all he has to do is pour it into the dog's bowl. No, he says that he knows that this is the way it should be done, because this is the way the dog likes it.

No harm, I guess, only I did not leave a container with one dog pill on the counter. It was the usual lunch-time container of kibble with two dog pills in it, all of it to be given to Annie. Now David doesn't recognize the plastic container or the pill, nor does he remember that he feeds the dog at lunchtime. Instead, David is convinced that I have left this lone pill on the counter to confuse him. He again complains about things being left all over the place.

I put something in the trash and see three medium-sized used coffee cups from Dunkin' Donuts. I ask David if he has had three coffees from Dunkin' Donuts today. He says no and by the way, would it at all be any of my business if he had?

I see that he has bought another snow shovel today. It's the wrong time of year to be buying snow shovels. I ask why he has bought another one. He says because he could not find the two shovels he bought yesterday. He asks, where did they go? What did I do with them? I told him that I had not touched them, that they are in the same spot where he put them. I open the door and show him the shovels to the left of the door. He says that he did not put them there. He blames me for moving things around. Everything is said in a forceful, loud, controlling tone of voice.

Later this same day, he brings me coffee. He is in a much better mood. In between, he has been out to walk the dogs and I have made dinner for him. I understand that he is starting to feel some insecurity in being alone and potentially doing something wrong.

✦ ✦ ✦ ✦ ✦ ✦

It was a good decision to pull David off the new medication, the Namendia. When Devon came over today, he was so excited because he got a baseball pitcher—the kind that automatically spits out the balls so that you can practice batting. We put it in the basement and Devon disappeared for quite a while, playing with it. David went down there awhile. A bit later, Devon came upstairs and told me in a very serious tone of voice that he needed to talk with me.

He took me into the bathroom and closed the door. He said very quietly that David had thrown a ball at him and hurt him. I asked him what he meant and what was this about? Didn't he mean the machine that pitched the ball out had hit him with a ball? No, he said, Papa *threw* the ball at him hard. "He did it twice." After a while, I got the story out that David had been playing with Devon with the pitching machine and had apparently gotten angry. He threw two balls directly at Devon, one striking his upper arm. I looked at Devon's arm and there found a large round red spot.

The worse injury was to Devon's spirit and emotions. He clearly could not fathom why his grandfather would do this to him. He put away the pitching machine and all of the balls and said he never wanted to play with it again. I had to try to explain to Devon that Papa has a sickness and that he was on the wrong medicine. He would be feeling better soon, but that we would have to watch over Papa a little more closely. He had not meant to hurt him.

I vow that I will not let this happen again.

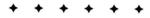

It has now been several weeks since David has been entirely off the Namendia pills and he has been in a much better mood. He is back to sleeping a lot and sleeping very late in the morning. He will routinely sleep 12 to 14 hours a night. While he has continued to show some aggressiveness and anger, it is not to the same level as before.

I often wish that I could recall even more of my observations about David during the day. There are hundreds of things that occur each day that define his illness. Generally, it's the absence of short-term memory and, perhaps because of that, a lack of focus that is very extreme. It is slowness and obsessiveness and repetitiveness. It is an individual sense of logic that does not make sense to other people. It is being easily overstimulated and it is difficulty processing information. This last symptom seems to be getting worse.

Yesterday, David called the shopping cart at Home Depot "the toboggan." I thought that was pretty creative. But he referred to Home Depot as "that big store over there." He asks or comments on the same things over and over within a few seconds or minutes of the previous comment. We went to the symphony last night and the first piece was by Verdi, the third piece by Mahler. While Verdi was on, David asked if this was Mahler. No, this is the Verdi. Thirty seconds later...this is the Mahler, right? No, this is the Verdi. A minute later, he says that he likes this piece by Mahler. No, I tell him again —this is the Verdi.

David had no problems driving to the symphony, but once there, he was agitated looking at the other cars parked around him. A van was parked outside of the lines. He kept looking at it and then looking at our car to try to figure it out. I told him, it was the van that was parked oddly, not our car. Our car was fine. He kept looking at the cars all around. I told him to get out and check it out if he was uncomfortable. He did. When he got back in, he decided to move our car to a different space.

Increasingly, things have to fit his sense of logic, which may not match my sense of logic. I try very hard to withhold my comments. I am sure they would come out sounding like criticisms. I don't want to be critical.

Leaving the parking lot after the symphony, David ran over a stone, which no one could have clearly seen. He took it personally, though, and made a quick right turn in the wrong direction. Home was the other way. When I told him gently that he was going the wrong way, he made some remark and then made a quick turn left into a parking lot, did a fast spin around and then gunned it back down in the other direction. I told him that he appeared agitated. He said he was trying to check the oil gauge while holding onto a thermos of coffee (which was fine without having to be held) and turn around all at the same time because of me. In other words, I should have just left him alone and everything would have been fine. These aggressive and agitated tendencies while driving worry me. I know I will have to take his keys away soon. If he can't drive, he certainly shouldn't be working.

Earlier in the day, he had been determined to arrange Kristin's garbage cans in the back of his truck just right. He took them out and rearranged them a number of times. They had to be arranged exactly right in order to not fall over. These were old empty cans that were going to be put in the dump, so it really didn't matter if they fell over, but it was very important to David to arrange the cans according to his sense of logic about them. I waited patiently until he was satisfied.

But it's April again and, against all odds, David is getting ready to return to work. He is just not ready to quit. He shouldn't be working or driving or cooking or even using half the tools we still have in the house and garage. How do I exert these controls over him?

Am I allowing him to be totally embarrassed by his diminished skills and logic? I certainly can't see him painting up all the buoys in any organized fashion. His uniforms are a mess. He keeps fighting me about buying new ones, seeing nothing wrong with big oil and grease spots.

Worse, am I allowing him to put other people in danger? His response times are slowed. What if there is an emergency? He is so easily distractible. What about the panic attacks he had last year? The people he works with must know that something is seriously wrong with him. How can they not know? Will they let him come back to work? Maybe I should I just let him be angry with me, take over and demand that I am now in charge of his life. I guess that's what I need to do. I have a pending sense of dread. I'm damned if I do and damned if I don't, and so is he.

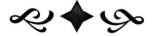

Then of course, when you think things can't get worse, they do. A few days after David returned to work, I fell off a retaining wall and landed with all my weight on the heel of my left foot, breaking my heel transversely across the bottom in a big nasty break that put me in a foot to knee cast. With my toes and knee swollen and everything in between in throbbing burning pain, I tried to hobble about on crutches and quickly found that I was severely limited. You cannot carry anything in your hands when you are on crutches. It's like losing three limbs.

Kristin came over and helped with meals for a few days. She even washed my toes for me. She soothed her dad and made sure he had his ice cream. That made him happy, if only for a short while. Lisa came down on the weekends and made me sit and do nothing while she tended to house cleaning and dishes.

For the rest of the time and over the course of seven weeks, I will have no choice but to depend on David's help or lack of it. Mostly he just doesn't want to deal with it. He groans and sighs and asks, "What else, your highness?" and tells me that all I do is bark out orders.

So, I sometimes sit and ask for nothing and nothing is what I get—nothing to drink or eat, no TV, no book, no shoe, no sock and no David. He is at the other end of the house. This past week, I think he has finally come to terms with the fact that life is very different now without me tending to all of his needs. We are both now doing the minimum to get out to work each morning and to feed ourselves each night. I have such an appreciation for older people and for handicapped people. Life becomes mostly about survival from day to day. You learn to appreciate all the details that you otherwise miss each day.

Sitting more now, I have more time to reflect. David's condition has gotten worse. At times, it seems that he simply slips quietly to the next higher level of this disease and I don't notice it at first until I add up several things that are different. Could he live without me? Right now, yes he could, but not up to my standards. There's an admission! My sense of normal sometimes feels so assaulted by his bedlam. We have been left to ourselves this week. One kitchen shade is jerked up diagonally across the window, while the other shade is pulled up to the top and out of sight. This must look lovely from the outside. There is a large kettle sitting on the stove, but I don't know why. Half a bottle of David's soda has been sitting on the counter all morning with the cover sitting beside it.

An unopened green plastic container of Quaker State Oil sits beside the soda on the counter. That was purchased a couple of weeks ago for the truck. I told David we would take the truck to Jiffy Lube, he did not have to change the oil any more. David protested that he had always changed the oil. Again, I told him not anymore—enjoy it, don't complain about it. Will I have to fight him over this?

A mix of clean and dirty dishes lines the counter by the sink. Quite often, David does not empty the dishwasher completely in order to start over with a new load of dirty dishes. He takes a few out, gets distracted, adds a few dirty dishes then closes the door. Later, he will open the door, notice the one or two dirty dishes and sigh about how many dishes we make, turning the dishwasher on to run again with its 95 percent clean load.

The garage is full of garbage. It was always David's job to go to the dump, but he no longer thinks about going to the dump. He has no sense of smell, so he does not notice the stink. It will just have to sit there because now I can't take it. The dogs have not eaten today. Sometimes, David can no longer manage the feeding process, which involves opening a can, getting the dishes, adding some dry food, mixing it up and apportioning it out to the two dogs. I have given David explicit instructions, a few words at a time. "Get the can from the shelf. Good, now get the large bowl from the top of the refrigerator. Okay, now get the smaller bowl that is on the floor over there..." Sometimes when I do this, he whips around at me—"Do you think I'm stupid?" or "Yeah, I know you think I'm seven years old."

He hands me a steaming cup of coffee when I am standing in the kitchen balancing on one foot with my hands on each crutch. I tell him thanks, but no thanks. I cannot carry a cup of coffee. He looks at me blankly. I repeat it and motion to my crutches. Then, he gets it.

It has been over a month since David returned to work. My injury has been a distraction up to now. We have had several discussions about his need to retire. Both his doctors, his regular doctor and his neurologist, advised him in April in no uncertain terms that he should not continue working, that he is 100 percent disabled. So I finally got serious about filling out his disability retirement application. It will be a long process, but it should be ready to file by next week. Meanwhile, David flip-flops between being insecure about work one day and confident the next. So far, there have been no boat trips, so there is not much to worry about. The weather has not been good for boating.

✦ ✦ ✦ ✦ ✦ ✦

Only a day later and we are already so different. David worked his last day today. Yesterday, he called me at work to come pick him up, because he had locked his car keys in his truck at work down near the dock. He got a ride back to the office, so I picked him up from the office and drove him back to the dock where his truck was parked. I had the spare key and handed it to him. He put it in the tray between the front seats of my car. When he got out of the car, he forgot to take the spare key with him. He thanked me and waved goodbye. In moments like these, I'm never sure if I should say something to try to help him or just watch it happen. If I try to help, he is often angry about me treating him like a little kid. If I don't help, I feel like I am letting him down, not being supportive.

Ultimately, David realized that he did not have the spare key and turned back, wondering where his own keys were. I had to remind him that he had locked them in the truck and that was, in fact, why I was there. I explained that I had given him my spare key to unlock the truck, but oh, look—there it is still in the tray between the seats! I hand it to him again and he successfully unlocks the truck door and gets in.

When David came home from work later that night, he was quiet and withdrawn, then became stressed and fitful. He put his head down on the table and said, "I can't do it. I can't do it anymore. I'm in a fog."

I wanted to dissolve to a heap on the floor, but instead put my arm around his shoulder while he explained that he had been upset that the pumpout motor was not working very well and he was unable to repair it. He had cleaned some of the corrosion, but believed that he had lost a part and that his boss would be very angry with him. We had fixed the 1st of July for his date of retirement, but I suggested that we move up his last day of work. Why couldn't he go out on sick leave now? David looked at me, lost, bewildered, finished and ever so thankful toward me for the suggestion. I hugged him and told him not to worry.

"Do you think I could? Could I do that?"

"Of course you can, David," I replied. "You are sick after all. Sick leave applies. You are too fatigued and stressed to go into work because you can no longer figure things out. That is just the way it is. You have to realize that you keep trying to do more than you are capable of doing."

This was a rare moment in which I could talk to David directly about his limitations. He seemed very relieved and asked me if I would go in and talk to his boss. I told him of course I would.

So, I did. I called his office requesting a day of sick leave and then I made an appointment with his boss. I used to work for the town and knew his boss, so this wasn't as strange as it sounds. In the meeting, I told his boss that I thought that he had treated David very well over the years, but that it was now time for David to retire. I explained that David would be applying for the town's disability. His boss was very supportive. He said that David had been honest with him about his problems, but very recently, it had become clear that David was now a safety threat. He was very glad that David had made the decision to retire and so he was now relieved of the burden of having to talk to him about his limitations. I requested sick leave for David until July 1 and then he would officially retire, with the disability application in the works.

And so it was done. David was effectively no longer employed. My heart ached for him.

✦ ✦ ✦ ✦ ✦ ✦

That night, I went home and finished up the last parts of David's retirement application and the next day, I hand-carried the doctor's statement form to his neurologist, certainly the most likely person to provide a disability certification.

The next day, I received a call from the neurologist's office and a message that I needed to call them. When I called, I was told that the neurologist would be providing his file notes, but would not write a statement. In fact, he did not "do statements." I was incredulous. How was that possible? There was a narrative part to the disability application. The most logical person to complete it would be David's neurologist. The form requested that the doctor treating the person for their condition should be the one to provide this statement. "No," the secretary said, "he won't do it. I don't know why. He just has a policy. He does not do these statements." I could feel my entire body reacting.

How was it possible that the very doctor who has been treating him for his illness for the past two years, who states that he is

100 percent disabled and that he should not be working, will not support him when it comes down to writing a statement? I asked to speak to the doctor.

"No," the doctor confirmed, "I won't complete a statement like that. It is a legal thing, and I will not write anything that can be used for legal purposes."

"No," I explained. "It is not a 'legal thing,' it's David's life and our ability to pay our bills. David does not qualify for Social Security Disability because he worked for a municipality. This is his only opportunity for a disability income. This is a state retirement system, and the application process is very detailed and demanding. Your statement is required."

Again, the doctor said that he would supply his notes, but he would not write a statement. He said that the notes would be enough. By now, I was crying on the phone with him. The most critical part of David's disability application was being denied by the doctor who was treating him. How did this make sense? The doctor explained that he had reviewed the form and found it to be "full of legalese and Massachusetts regulations." A case review and legal opinion would be required. He simply did not do case reviews. There could be information that could be used against him, he said. What if something had already happened in David's job, for example, and he could be accused of being able to prevent it by telling David sooner that he should not be working. I would have to get an attorney to explain every word on the form to him. Even after that, he would not be likely to fill in any written statement. "They can have my records, but that's all. I am not writing a statement."

A few minutes later, I received a call from David's primary-care doctor. Apparently the neurologist was at least bothered enough by my reaction to call him and offer him up as an alternative. David's primary-care doctor was almost as astonished as I was at the neurologist's lack of direct support, but he would have no problem writing the needed statement. He wrote it and faxed it to me the same day.

It's a 20-page application that has now been signed, co-signed, copied and submitted. I am waiting for various medical records to be sent to the retirement board, but with many phone calls, everything necessary has finally been filed on David's behalf.

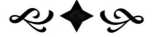

We are now seeing significantly more negativism, anger and childish behavior since David officially "retired." He complains so much and is so mean at times that I have to get away from him. I feel so much the depths of my depression that I am afraid that I won't find my way back.

I have now accepted that his total lack of empathy and understanding during these past many weeks is disease-induced behavior. This has been difficult to accept, but somewhere in my reading, I did find this can be a symptomatic trait of Alzheimer's Disease. He is so focused on himself that he has no ability to consider the needs or feelings of others. It is otherwise disgustingly egocentric behavior, which is what makes it so hard to accept. Somehow, I am supposed to set aside my own personal feelings.

Over the past two weeks, I have been told that I am not to be believed, I am a liar and a hypocrite. I have been told that I treat him like a slave, that I steal his time. When I ask for help, I am told to get up and get things myself. I have also been told that I could have retired too if that was what I wanted, so I should go out to work and support him until I can provide the same retirement income that he has for himself. I'm thinking that, since I never worked for the military, that should take me about 20 years!

I continue to sit with my broken foot, waiting for the cup of coffee that will never come and the empathy that he cannot feel.

✦ ✦ ✦ ✦ ✦ ✦

To somehow take care of David and take care of me at the same time, I have had to learn to make do. My foot still cannot bear the slightest bit of weight, so I pulled a knapsack out of my closet and strapped it onto my back to fill with the day's newspapers, magazines and even dirty dishes to take back to the kitchen. Kristin and Dennis bought me a little red wagon that is very cute and very practical. I can pile two plates of food, silverware and glasses and pull it behind me to bring our meals to the table in the den where we eat. When David is right in front of me, he can be helpful. I can hand him the water jug and ask him to take it to the table. He will do that, but might balk at taking it back to the refrigerator for me when our meal is done.

The grass is growing and I can't mow it, but Lisa will be down on the weekend so she will help. I have to let go of all those standards. Things can no longer be perfect.

I am on my way to work at the main office today, but I am so tired. I watch as coffee drips from my thermos onto my nice green jumper. I am able to wipe away the excess liquid in each drop, but cannot wipe away the spots. Another drip, another spot. I watch but feel nothing. It's been six long weeks of having a broken foot and trying to hobble around on crutches. The crutches steal the use of my hands. Add David to the mix and the chores multiply and expand to fill every waking moment of the day.

The leaky thermos drips little drops of fatigue onto me and I am too tired to have an opinion. So, I watch.

✦ ✦ ✦ ✦ ✦ ✦

We seem to be back to an extreme version of the winter layoffs when David used to sit in the kitchen doing not much more than kitchen things all winter. Now that he is in a permanent layoff situation, it is much the same and yet much different. It is hot summer and yet when David gets up this morning, he will put on his long-sleeved flannel shirt and long pants. He will stand in the kitchen and look around much like he used to do, but it is for a longer period of time. He will stare out the window, sometimes carefully studying and re-positioning items on the counter. Most days he will remember to take his morning pill. Some days he does not. He will pour himself a cup of coffee and continue to look around.

He will make some loving comment to the dogs like "Good girl" to Annie or "Aren't you a handsome guy!" to little Ipo. He will pick up Ipo and walk around with him. Eventually, he will sit down at the table, pick up some of his special pens and work on the day's crossword, usually getting five across and four down or maybe four across and five down. He is fixed at this odd percentage of his prior 100 percent crossword success rate. He will let the dogs out and stand waiting for them outside their fence, then he will let the dogs in. He will go find the cat, hold it for a while even if it squirms, then he will put the cat out and sit back down to his crossword. Two hours will pass by in this way.

He will then look at his list for the day, using a special marker to fill in the check blocks on completed items. Some days he does well with his list, other days he does not. Yesterday, he checked one item, "Take AM pill." He vacuums using the big vacuum then forgets we have a big vacuum and uses the little bare floor sweeper on the rugs. When I say that he should use the big one, intended for rugs, he asks how would I know.

"The little vacuum is a piece of junk anyway. It used to be great, but now it's like everything else around here—broken."

"Yes," I say. "Because you keep using it on the rugs. It's supposed to be used on bare floors."

"And why would that be?" he remarks. "Do you think vacuums have rules? Where is the rule book?"

"Yes, they have instructions and that one's instructions said to use it on the bare floor. You can choose to believe me or not." *Why am I persisting in doing this?*

"I don't believe you. Why would I believe you?" he asks sarcastically. Of course, I deserve the sarcasm. I just don't know when to quit. He gives up on vacuuming, puts the vacuum in the corner for the day. He returns to the kitchen and carefully prepares two Toaster Strudels. Later in the day, he will eat a couple of Little Debbie donuts and throughout the day, fill mug after mug with coffee. He keeps a large kettle on the stove to pour in hot coffee so it has the proper surface area to cool so that he can have iced coffee later. Now I know why he keeps that big kettle on the stove. I was wondering what he was doing with it. Yesterday, he emptied the coffeepot into the kettle, then wiped out the pot with a white towel. He could not figure out why this white towel was now brown.

"It's from the coffee," I explain.

"What coffee?"

"The coffee in the pot." I tell him. "Remember you had coffee in the pot?" I have to learn not to start so many sentences with "Remember." Of course he doesn't "remember"!

"Why is this brown?" he asks again.

"Because of the coffee, David. You did not wash the pot. You dried it out with that towel."

"Oh, I guess I thought I washed it."

"Do you know where this is from?" David asks. He is pointing to the brown coffee stain on the towel.

"No," I reply. "You know, I might have dropped it on the floor. Sorry. I should have put it in the wash." Sometimes it's just easier to tell a white lie and get the subject finished.

"Oh," David says. He seems satisfied.

I leave the room.

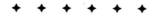

The summer has moved on and we have been consumed by getting ready for the sale of our old house—finally. The first offer to purchase did not go through, so we have waited now another nine months for a new buyer. I have never been more stressed worrying about the double mortgages I have taken on to accomplish this move, combined with our loss of income from David's job. I began to doubt that my decision to buy first, get David re-situated and then worry later about selling our old house was the right thing to do. Surely, David was suffering miserably from my stress, so in the end, I'm not sure that I saved him from any discomfort by doing things this way.

What we had left behind at the old house and outbuildings was quite a bit more than it seemed. As we filled truckload after truckload, David was very angry at times about having to clean out and give away things that he had defined his life around. We would have a good day, then a bad day. A bad day is more and more filled with David's growing anger and resentment that can get a little scary at times. There were moments where he literally seethed in anger and could not let go of the feeling. I wished that I could have left him out of it, but I needed his muscles. Although my foot is on the mend, it is still difficult for me to walk, particularly carrying heavy boxes.

We have been notified by the state retirement board that David has a hearing before a three-doctor panel at the end of the month. We have to travel to Middleboro, about 60 miles away. There are two orthopedic doctors and one neurologist. I don't know what to think about that. I guess they must hear a lot of cases involving mobility issues. I am already feeling intimidated on David's behalf.

David is worried about what he should say to them. I told him that he might not have to say anything, but if he did have to comment, it should be to say that he knows that he cannot do his job anymore because of this illness. The more direct I try to be, the more difficult it becomes to try to talk to David in a way that gains his acceptance. By the night before the hearing, he is quite convinced that he is ready to go back to work and wonders if they will let him do that. I didn't want to put words in his mouth but said, "David, that is ridiculous! You are not working because you cannot do the job because you have an illness. You know that if you cannot do the job 100 percent, then you can be a danger, and I know that you don't want to hurt other people. It is really okay for people with an illness to say that they cannot do a job anymore when they are too ill to do the job. You are too ill to do the job! The town would be liable for anything that you do wrong. I just can't see that you are okay with being in that situation. I don't think that you would want something bad to happen."

"Okay." David said that he understood, but I wasn't sure.

In fact, the doctors turned out to be less threatening than I had presumed, but David was still quite stressed by the whole experience.

When we arrived, the doctors were going in and out of a meeting room with an open door. They seemed a bit jovial, talking with each other about family things. After a while, I could overhear them talking about their next case, which of course was David. "Well," one doctor said, "this case is really all about the paper. We won't have to do much talking to him." "No," said another doctor, "I'll just ask him a few questions and that should do it."

Interestingly, though, when they got David in the small room with them, with me at his side, it seemed that they could not ask enough questions. They were very interested. The case was interesting and sad, and you could read that in their eyes.

Here was an apparently very healthy, good-looking and still relatively young-looking man with bright eyes and a smiling face, anxious to please. Yet, David did not know what town he was in. He could not remember the name of the former president but he did remember who he was by remarking, "Oh, yes, that asshole. What he did (Lewinsky)... I hate him." Apparently the doctors readily agreed with him and laughed heartily.

When David was given the names of three prior presidents and was asked to choose the one who had preceded President Clinton, he could not match the name with the person he knew as the former president, even with gentle prodding and two chances. He remembered his own daughters' names, but he could not do simple math. One of the doctors turned to me and asked, "So, you said that you still work. When you go to work, is it all right to leave him home alone?" Of course, I knew at that moment that the doctors would be supporting David's claim.

As we were going out to the car, one of the doctors walked up to me with a sympathetic look. He said, "It must be very..." then he caught himself. "Uh, well...." He knew he shouldn't be talking to me. They are supposed to be an impartial panel. Yet how could they be impartial in a case like this? How could anyone be impartial? Impossible.

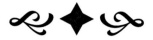

David's disability claim was approved and I am giddy with excitement. In this life where lack of control rules the day, I feel I have won. It means that we will be getting just under $1,000 a month to help with our finances and it is such a relief now that David is no longer working. We had lost not only David's seven months of pay, but also the unemployment compensation that he used to receive for the other five months of the year. So little and yet so much. So necessary. While this was not as much as he would have received for Social Security Disability compensation, I was ecstatic to be able to move some of the financial worries off my radar screen.

Today, though, we have had another full day of anger. This has been happening more and more. The day after our trip to Middleboro, David had a very, very angry day. He could not be approached. His face was screwed up with hard frown lines. It seems that something has changed with him, from deep within him, so that I am not sure day-to-day what his mood will be like. Today, he got up at 11:00, ate no food, then started incessantly cleaning. For two hours, he cleaned like a crazy person. He could not be approached, had a very hard edge and a very angry face…the kind of face that says, *I mean business; stay away if you value your life!*

In this dark and angry mood, David typically makes very mean remarks to me in an effort to make me angry too. He alluded to the cleaning he used to do in the military, indicating that this was a special skill and of course, it is. He can be quite a good house cleaner, quite a good dish washer, quite a good clothes folder. On this day, I found him in the bathroom with a large bath towel and five dish towels totally soaked with water. I asked him what he was doing with the towels. He barked out, "What does it matter? What could it possibly matter to you? Why should you have anything to say about it?"

He knew I had been cleaning downstairs in the basement and he referred to my cleaning as "playing around." How many bags of garbage did I have to show for my work? I told him that I had eight. "That's all? That's all you did? Is all that shit gone now?" I slunk off. It's no use approaching him when he is like this and even if I try to coax him away with a cup of coffee or offer of lunch, his attention cannot be diverted from the task at hand. It's on his agenda to be angry today.

I waited a while and then, in the early afternoon, I asked him to go to the beach. It's a beautiful fall day and the trees are an explosion of color. It's the time of year when people on Cape Cod reclaim their beaches. There are no worries about crowds or parking. You can revel in the sounds of the surf and pretend that no one actually owns waterfront property. But David said no, a resounding "NO," carrying on in his dedicated angry mode. He was now angry that he could not find any of his hats. Eventually he found one, calling it a "piece-of-shit-hat" as he went out the door to mow the lawn one last time for the season. Annie, the big black lab, went in the closet and stayed there for most of the day.

I went to the beach by myself.

✦ ✦ ✦ ✦ ✦ ✦

It is becoming harder and harder for me to relate to David and his illness. It's beginning to define who he is. I am forgetting the David I married and that makes me angry. So we are two angry people trying to live together. It's not working well.

I realize that I am particularly bothered by any perception that David is just fine. It happens or I read into it that it happens, and then I am angry that other people cannot see what I see every day. A friend of mine saw David in the store. She told me that they talked about the end of the boating season, the fall weather, how great it was that the summer people were off the beaches and roads giving us our beautiful Cape Cod back again. She remarked about how much shopping David was doing, how well David looked and what a nice conversation they had.

I wanted to respond, *Well, good for you. You are obviously doing better than me. I can't talk to him at all anymore. We never seem to have a nice conversation anymore.* It was as though she had said, *What on earth are you talking about that David has Alzheimer's Disease? He is well enough to go do your shopping, isn't he? He seems normal enough to me, so why do you always say that you have to hurry home to take care of him? Maybe you're the one who is sick. If he's well enough to drive and go shopping, then he must be just fine. You just expect too much, don't you? You just can't be satisfied, can you?*

What I'm really feeling is that I am not up to this task of being a caregiver. I am a facts-and-figures kind of girl. I like to be direct and clear. I like to plan things so well that nothing, not even a whisker, can bend the wrong way for fear that I will snap it back like a rubber band. I like order and logic. I certainly don't like Alzheimer's Disease!

I am never sure that I am doing enough or responding in a supportive way, but I keep trying. I have just reduced my work schedule. While it's only a reduction of five hours a week, it will be five hours a week more that I can spend at home with David. I explained to my supervisor that nothing really dangerous is going on, nothing really harmful. Then I was mad at myself for characterizing it that way. What am I talking about? I live in Crazyville. No, it's not harmful. It's just crazy and I have to somehow maintain my sanity in Crazyville. How to explain it? All I could say was "I'm finding that I need to be there more often to supervise David." My supervisor and my coworkers are very supportive. They have a pretty good idea about what I am dealing with.

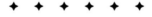

I'm standing in the Crazyville garage, trying to decide if there is any way that I can put it to rights for the winter. I've started to bring in the plastic lawn furniture and the bird bath and hoses. The spreader is still stuck with lime, and a large empty bag of lime and lime dust is strewn beside it. We used to have a nice lawn, but it is now turning more yellow and brown than I have ever seen before. I just can't keep up with David. He doesn't always tell me what he is going to do before doing it and before I know it, he is off doing something he shouldn't be doing. This was enough lime to do four of our front yards, but David decided that our lawn needed lots and lots of lime this year so he dialed up the spreader to 12 and loaded it on. No wonder the grass isn't green anymore!

I make a mental note that the lawn mower will certainly need a trip to the Sears repair center in the spring for a makeover. It sits silent now, but this year it had to be a real soldier. David had some trouble starting the mower this year. I would listen for the poor mower to try to start, to cough and sputter, stop and then try to start again as David pulled and pulled on the cord. I would run out and try some weak, half-hearted suggestion to see if he would take the bait. "David, if you try it this way, pushing the primer button three times (as it says in the directions printed right on the frame), maybe it would respond better. What do you think? Can we try it this way?" Sometimes he would let me try. Other times he would make a derisive comment about what I think I know.

Yesterday, David went to the dump as he always does every weekend. Good for him. He can still do that. He has a big truck that could perhaps hold 20 bags of garbage. Yet here I am planning to go to the dump again today. I feel so robbed of my time. He has left two bags behind and one is the most aromatic of them all. It's the bag of dog shit. No nice way to say it. It is the bag with the doggie doos that David has responsibly collected into Ziploc bags while on his walks with the dogs. He used to deposit them right into the kitchen trash bin until I went berserk. I would be overcome with the smell as soon as I came into the house each night. But David? He smelled nothing at all. So they get moved to the garage and then on to the dump each week, unless David forgets.

Then there is the other garbage can full of wet, moldy, smelly grass. David has his rituals and one ritual he has adopted is that when he mows the lawn or rakes the lawn, he dumps the clippings directly into the garbage cans without benefit of a plastic liner. He would never have done this years ago. But then he can't smell it and this is the way that it makes sense to him. I have to go get the box of plastic liners and dump the clippings into the bags, and then if I don't wash out the cans they will continue to stink. I am the cleanup girl. I wanted to read a book today. It's Sunday.

At the very back of the garage is all my gardening stuff, now covered with stuff David has laid on top of it—utility electric cords, a saw, rope, wire, boat parts, a hammock. He has pushed the contents of the garage back to the back of the garage so tightly that I can no longer reach my gardening tools. Is this on purpose? I don't know.

As I move into the hallway inside the side door, I see that David's car keys are not hung up. It may take him half a day to find his keys and I will be called into the search if I'm home. On the shelf are his pills that I have correctly dosed out into little trays and a bottle of pills waiting to remind me to order a refill. There is a dog-and-cat food shelf, with the food organized by day. This was a most wonderful Christmas gift from Kristin last year. She painted each shelf "Monday," "Tuesday," and so on. It's the only way to know if the animals have been fed or not. If the shelf is empty, hopefully the answer is "Yes." I fill up some of the empty shelves with the remaining cans so we can be sure that the dogs and cat get fed on each day of the week.

In the utility closet, there are piles of Ziploc bags stuffed into every nook and cranny. These are the bags that David uses to collect the doggie doos when he walks the dogs. They are turned inside out and readied for the walk, but when David goes out the door, he always takes new bags out of the Ziploc boxes. He never takes the bags he has prepared. Consequently, we probably have 100 Ziploc bags turned inside out in the closet plus two boxes of unopened Ziplocs. We also have the cleaning products that David can't remember to put back under the sink. There are also now several of David's jackets hanging in the closet. He was complaining that he had no coat, so I got all the winter clothes out and arranged his closet, his dresser and this rack in the utility room so that he could easily see that he had clothes to wear. He should be able to find his things easily now. Should. Wishful thinking on my part, I guess.

On the hat rack, though, there are none of David's ball caps. He has always had five to 10 at any one time to choose from. Where have they gone? They are all missing. No matter how hard I try to organize and keep up with David, I just can't seem to keep up.

On the kitchen counter are the wet towels. There are always wet towels. He uses them to clean up the counters. I think he no longer remembers that we have paper towels or what they are used for. He will no longer use a sponge for anything but he has a reason for that, because sponges carry bacteria. The dishwashing liquid must be placed under the sink. The hand washing liquid must stay on the window sill. That's the way he likes it. If I change it, he will change it back. It's okay. I'm getting used to this.

In with the coffee cups I find a bag of Chex Mix. I put it back with the snack foods alongside David's three boxes of Captain's Choice Variety Pack crackers. His boxes of Little Debbies are sometimes in the snack cabinet and sometimes in the refrigerator. I won't mess with these. They can stay wherever they find a home. In the refrigerator, there are three remaining bottles of Zazz soda, flavored soda water without any sugar or sweetener. I like them too, but David usually fills the refrigerator with them, buying 10 bottles at a time. He believes that the refrigerator works better when you fill it up. So, he fills it up, then he gets angry when I have to take a few out of the vegetable drawer to put in some actual vegetables.

I have tried to hide the scouring powder. The Formica countertops have been scoured so much they are scratched and dull, but David believes that Formica is hardy and he can scour it as much as he wants and he can set down the hot coffeepot on it. When I show him the marks, he says that they were there all along.

He will not put a frying pan in the sink. The only way to clean a frying pan, he says, is to clean it out with salt and a paper towel. Sometimes, I have to scour the frying pan when he is not looking, in order to use it again. Sometimes the coffee tastes like soap. Luckily I usually notice that right away. Always, there are dirty cups in the cupboard from David having unloaded a dirty dishwasher. I'm used to it by now. I always rinse out any cup that I take from the cupboard to use.

Crazyville. There is some craziness in every room.

This is my life now.

✦ ✦ ✦ ✦ ✦ ✦

It's 9:45 a.m. and David is asleep. I love this time on the weekend. I am alone and able to think. Most nights, David follows me around and waits up for me. He will prepare the coffeepot, or pretend to be organizing newspapers or put a cup in the dishwasher... anything to wait for me to go to bed. I seem to want to stay up later and later and end up dozing off in the den. We are so drifting apart hour by hour and minute by minute.

I am tired, and when I am this tired, I have to leave off writing for a while. I want so much to be a better person, a better caregiver, a better wife. But it just seems to be more of the same, more of the same, more of the same.

In reality, I know I am a bitter, angry and negative person. Some of that rubbed off of David and onto me, and so this disease has changed me as well. I just can't protect myself from it. Much of the rest of it is born of the resentment that I feel.

Year Four

Well, it's the beginning of January and this is the beginning of my fourth year of recording notes and thoughts about David and about me. As I gathered my files together to put under one subdirectory this year, I was struck by the fact that both progress and decline have been so slow. This could literally be three years ago, except...except for what?

A few things are quite distinctly different and many other things are only vaguely different. One thing that is new is that David cannot take his medications by himself any longer. He cannot determine what day of the week it is. Now, even looking at the newspaper gives no clue. He cannot remember what he reads and I'm beginning to think that the textual words are beginning to lose their meaning. He may read "Sunday," but by the time he moves from the den to the little shelf in the kitchen where he keeps his pills, he has already lost the word "Sunday."

It really doesn't matter anyway, because he can no longer associate the weekday with the letters on his pill box, "S M T W T F S." That must confuse other people as well. He keeps trying, but it ends up with confusion, missed pills on some days, double pills on other days.

So, I open the little containers and walk his pill over to him where he opens his mouth and sticks out his tongue obediently for me to put the pill on his tongue. Why he wants to act like a child, I don't know, but I don't fight him on this and dutifully put the little pill on his tongue. He is taking 10 milligrams of Aricept and 20 milligrams of paroxetene (Paxil) to help with his moods, and there he stays. The doctor upped his Aricept to 15 milligrams, with the result that David became absolutely manic. He could not slow down or stop. He would vacuum

151

the same room over and over, walk the dogs, come back in and vacuum all over again. I decided to back him down to where he was previously, and although he has retained some of his manic behavior, it is better now, more manageable. Again, I am playing doctor, but then so is his doctor. It seems like we are always tweaking his medications.

Another change is that David has had some episodes of falling or jerking hard enough to cause him to drop what is in his hands, fall against the counter, spill coffee all over the floor, scrape his arm on the counter. I have not witnessed these episodes, but have come upon him right afterwards. A few days ago, he blamed the area rug we have in the kitchen, so I taped it down. He was convinced that the little carpet was the problem and did not remember falling anywhere else. David shared this new development with our Alzheimer's Support Group, and the fact that he talked about it independently told me that he felt it was significant.

Some days, David oddly gets up at 6:00 a.m., looking bleary-eyed and determined, as though he has something very important to do that day, but he cannot figure out what it is. Most days, though, he is like clockwork, now sleeping 13 hours straight.

I am still resentful. That hasn't changed. I still find it difficult to react to David with the understanding that he has an illness. If I stay home from work, he never asks if I'm home because I'm sick. If I come home early from work, he wouldn't know because he does not know my work hours. He does not know if I am early or late and he never asks. I truly believe that this is not about memory; it's about the absence of caring. While

I understand that this is also part of the disease process, it's a much sadder symptom than the loss of memory. I know that this is not directed at me personally. I know that. I know that. I know that. I just need to convince my heart of that.

✦ ✦ ✦ ✦ ✦ ✦

Tonight, we are not talking to each other. We have just had a war of words that is something evil and disgusting. I just will not be verbally abused and take it. I have to fight back despite the interference of this disease. I know this is my own weakness, but I just can't help it.

David saw my Walkman radio with headphones on the little table by my elliptical machine.

"There it is," he sputters. "You had it. You took it. All this time that I lost it and you had it this whole time."

"No, that's not yours. That's mine."

"Oh, sure, it's yours. Right, it's yours. So this just turns up and it's yours." His tone is so sarcastic.

"Yes, that's right, it *is* mine. It's my exercise radio."

"Why haven't I seen it before? You expect me to believe that story?"

"Yes, that's my radio, not your radio."

I go upstairs and David follows me. He is staring at me, challenging me. I know that he has this radio on the brain now.

He has accused me of thievery before, and this seems like much the same level of absurd gravity. I can feel it coming.

"Sure it's *your* radio. Sure. My radio has been missing and suddenly it turns up again and you call it your radio. You expect me to believe that when I haven't ever seen your radio before now?"

"I don't *call* it my radio. It *is* my radio. It's from my exercise bag, which is why you have not seen it before."

"Oh, really."

"Yes, really. It's been in my exercise bag for three years. I took it to the gym for two years straight, and for the last year, it has sat in the bag on the shelf in my closet. I took it out recently to use it when I exercised on the elliptical machine." I didn't mention the fact that the reason my gym bag had been idle for a year was that I could no longer fit in going to the gym when I was so preoccupied with caring for him. This fact just loaded my victim gun a little more. There was so much that David didn't know.

"You really are cunning. You used to have integrity, but now the real you shines through."

"I will not accept you calling me a liar. You can get your own dinner. I am done." And with that, I left the room, went to the spare bedroom and locked myself in for a while.

Of course, I couldn't bring myself to follow through with not providing dinner for David. Well, not exactly. Later, I came back out, put a frozen dinner in the oven, cooked it, took it out and put it on the table with a note beside it—"Yours" with an arrow. I ate my frozen dinner alone in front of the TV, watching a black-and-white movie from the '50s. The movie was a story about true love. *Very fitting*, I thought.

What cannot be communicated clearly about this exchange is the venom that comes spewing out of David's mouth when he talks. It is truly venomous. He has such a deep-seated hatred of me that it is on the edge of scary at times.

I cannot seem to stop my natural inclination to fight back. Why do I do this? I not only ignite his anger, I don't know when or how to stop it. My confidence as a caregiver is at an all-time low. This is just not the job for me. I have become David's worst enemy instead of his best friend.

David's tone is biting, searing, stinging, and cruel. My tone is often repetitious and monotonous to the point of making me sick. This constant fighting is the part that I am not so sure that I can survive for too long. The rest of it is almost minor by comparison.

Yet, each day there seems to be something new to deal with. David picks up all the dog dishes including the water dish and puts them in the dishwasher, but sometimes the dishwasher is not run for a day. Meanwhile, the dogs have no water. This would be unthinkable only a few years ago. David would never have let the dogs go without water for even half an hour. If I had ever done that, he would have screamed at me for being a total moron. This is beyond correcting. I cannot address this problem with him. It would result in another verbal altercation, and I have had enough of those for now. I will just have to keep a watch on the dogs' water dish.

✦ ✦ ✦ ✦ ✦ ✦

This is now a typical situation when I serve dinner. David gets up to get a fork. He comes back with a bowl. He comes back with the bag of salad. He comes back with the salt. He comes back with another glass. At some point, he realizes that he cannot eat without the fork and successfully gets the fork. I don't interfere, partly because I don't want to embarrass him or somehow diminish him because of his limitations. I want him to be successful. I also don't want him to be angry with me for interfering. All of this, though, is starting to be a tough balancing act.

I remark about the seven boxes of Toaster Strudels taking up so much room in the freezer. David says he did not buy them. Well, he corrects himself. He did buy some of them, but certainly not the four strawberry cream cheese ones because he does not like that kind! He doesn't know who keeps buying them. It's crazy, he says! I tell him that I do not eat them and do not buy them. He responds once again that he did not buy them, particularly not *that* kind that he doesn't like. This was several days ago. Just yesterday, when we were at the store together, I silently took out of our shopping cart the two strawberry cream cheese Toaster Strudels that David put in the cart to buy, yet again. I was smiling over that one. He did not notice that I took them out of the cart.

I guess I'm finally learning some stealthy approaches.

David has four pairs of black leather or leather-like winter gloves in his dresser. I keep urging him to put them in the closet with his coat, but he does not want to put them there. He says he is the guy who has to carry things and so he has to wear work gloves instead. He cannot wear his nice gloves. I tell him that he is not always carrying things and he should be wearing his black winter gloves. No, he cannot get his nice gloves dirty, so he will not wear them. So, when we are going out the door to dinner, he is wearing his industrial-strength blue canvas work gloves. This has to be okay because I just have to learn to choose my battles.

He carries my little dog "Ipo" everywhere. "Come on, little feller. Come on." Then he giggles incessantly.

I think I am going insane.

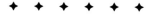

Kristin took David to the grocery store and later told me she was shocked at how often her dad would get very close to women in the store, particularly the clerks. He would greet each one like a long-lost friend. Some were friendly and others were stand-offish, to the point where Kristin felt that they were quite uncomfortable. David reached around a clerk to get something off the shelf and put a hand on her shoulder. It was clearly inappropriate. Kristin was upset and told me not to allow him to go shopping alone. I tried talking to David about it, but he accused Kristin of spying on him.

Now, I am trying to arrange joint shopping trips at least once a week, like a nice outing for us. If he only knew that it is glorified babysitting on my part; not only that, it keeps David off the road because I do the driving. If I send David off for something in the store, it will occupy him for 20 minutes and he will come back without the item he was sent to look for. Sometimes he gets mad at me for continuing to shop or moving so fast. I just give him something else to go look for.

Again, I am learning new approaches.

✦   ✦   ✦   ✦   ✦   ✦

Okay, now I am really angry. Of course, I've been angry for a while but that has been a simmering kind of anger. This is a bigger kind of anger. I cannot get hold of myself. Again, I am never quite sure how much this illness is responsible for and how much is David's own laziness, lack of attention and/or lack of caring. Ever-present now seems to be his jealousy and paranoia directed against me.

Yesterday, he said he wanted to apologize about the radio incident a week ago, because after all, it was only a radio and not worth arguing about.

"So I want to tell you I love you and I'm sorry about the radio."

I just stared at him, then I said, "No. The point is, I did not steal your radio and I will not accept being blamed and thought of as a dishonest person by you. I just won't accept it. And by the way, do you remember that?"

"What?"

"You remember that you accused me of stealing your radio a week ago? You really remember that?" I ask.

"Of course. Why wouldn't I?" he replies.

"Ah, because you have memory problems, and you don't remember anything else that happened in the last few days."

"Oh, no, that's not true. I remember lots of things."

Okay, I am the one who is now going crazy, I think. *Does he now have selective memory? Maybe he has intermittent Alzheimer's Disease?*

Since that exchange, he has glared at me over so many things that I've lost track. He lost a glove and kept coming into the kitchen remarking about his lost glove and looking straight at me. This is his version of accusing. He can say he is not accusing me, but when he comes into the same room where I am and remarks about everyone always taking his things while looking straight at me, there is not much left to the imagination. It seems to happen daily now, and some days (like this one), it seems to happen all day long.

I'm thinking that the reason he is angry with me over a missing glove is because a few days ago, I had told him that he should be wearing his nice gloves when we went out to dinner. I realize that it's not the missing glove that is making him angry. It's that the word *glove* is linked to a resentment that he still feels about my telling him what to do. I try to think back to exactly what I said to him. *Did I sound like a parent telling a child what to do?* Probably. And now it has turned into a vengeance attack against me.

While he was looking for his glove in the bedroom, I saw him holding his large stainless thermos. It was one of those idiotic scenes. He was bent over his nightstand holding his stainless thermos. Why does he have that in the bedroom? He always loved his thermos when he used to go to work. It was special to him. It dawns on me that he thinks I'm going to take it away from him. It's about loss, so many losses for him.

When he is not looking, I go into the bedroom to see where he has stashed the thermos and find, in his bottom dresser drawer, the box of Girl Scout cookies he bought today when we went out. I don't like cookies and wouldn't eat these, but still, he does not want me to take them. He does not want to lose them. I place them back in the drawer. So sad. I'm so sad.

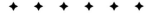

Every few days, it seems that we have a new object that has gone MIA. It immediately fuels a new argument. Where are his car keys? Did I take his keys? Why did I move his keys? Why did I have to touch his keys? Didn't I understand how important it is that I not move his things?

Well, I admitted to picking up his keys from the counter, thinking I was helping him by hanging them up; unfortunately, I put them on the wrong hook and, in so doing, learned a big lesson. Even moving something to a very logical place in my world of normal can be a very illogical place in his world of normal. I had placed the keys on a hook five inches away from the hook where David usually places his keys. Just that five-inch difference turned his world upside down. He could not find his keys. So now he is angry with me again, or maybe still.

I realize that I am trying to minimize the importance of these little things because the big things that I have to deal with are so big that I just don't have room for the little things. I see his overreactions as evidence of his weird, developing possessiveness that makes finding an object more important than loving and caring for me. On the periphery, I can appreciate to some degree that he is clinging to these very familiar things to maintain their familiarity for as long as possible. For me, though, the emphasis is in the wrong place. I want him to love me and trust me, to trust my care. I don't want him to be mad at me all the time for inadvertently moving things around. I wish these little things were not so important to him.

✦ ✦ ✦ ✦ ✦ ✦

Last week, David was complaining about the exercise machine being in the study and sitting too close to his desk.

"I didn't know all these people were going to be in there. How can I work at my desk with all these people and that machine crowding my desk?"

"Well, Kristin moved the exercise machine into the study because she wants to watch TV while she comes over to exercise, and right now, the TV is in the study. Once I finish painting the family room, I'll move it back in there," I explain.

In fact, the elliptical machine wasn't crowding David's desk at all, but it must have seemed that way to him. It was another change and he didn't like it one bit. I so much want to add, "You know you never even use that desk. I set it up for you with the computer, your paper, your special pens and even your music, but you never use it, so why would you care where I put the exercise machine?" Somehow, I restrain myself.

I put David's stereo in the study so he could listen to the music that he likes. Now he is angry about that too. He doesn't want his stereo in the study; he wants it in the workshop where he works.

This seemed ludicrous to me. Why would he want his nice old stereo system in the workshop with concrete walls and floors and sawdust and cobwebs all around? I was hurt because it had taken me so long to figure out how to connect all the wires to the various old system components and speakers. This job was clearly beyond his skills and he so missed his music after we moved. I thought that by setting up his stereo system in the study, I would have made him deliriously happy.

Not so.

What I didn't realize was that his comfort zone is now in the workshop and not in the study, and so that's where he wants his music, in the workshop where he likes to sit. That should be okay with me. Why isn't it okay with me?

I think it's because I am so unwilling to accept his losses. He cannot write anymore. He cannot use the computer anymore.

Obviously, he is not comfortable in the study, but this is especially sad to me. David had been such a PC fan right from the start, from the mid-'80s on. He had ordered a Hyperion from Canada, one of the earliest and coolest home PC systems. Then he bought a Lisa, another system for the PC adventurer. Then we got one of the first XTs and moved on through the familiar series of IBM-based systems. With every new PC that came along, David was right there in line waiting to purchase it. He had to be current with the latest technology. It fascinated him. He loved the Internet and spent years developing an expertise in genealogical research, tracing his family's roots back for centuries. *Now those skills are all gone? How can that be? Wasn't he still looking up things on the Internet just last year?*

Where did that David go? Now he sits in the workshop for hours. He likes to move around tools and boxes of screws and nails. There is a large table top near the washer and dryer. David can spend hours at that table folding clothes. *Why isn't that okay with me?*

Why does it take me so long to appreciate what he needs and to respond to his needs without this overwhelming anger?

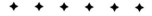

I am practicing my cello. Dedicated practice time is getting to be a rare commodity for me. David comes in, interrupting me with a scowling look on his face, glaring at me and holding a plastic card from our insurance company. The card has my name at the top and a list of contact phone numbers.

"Sure," he says, "*you* have a card. Where is *my* card?"

"What?"

"Why do you get a card and I don't have a card?"

"You do have a card." I get up, put down my cello, go out to the kitchen and retrieve his card from a shelf. "Here it is." I hand him the card.

"Well, what's it doing there? What good is it to put it there and not tell me about it? That's stupid for you to put it there. What good is it to me when I don't know it's there?" By this time he is yelling at me.

In my opinion, this is a stupid little plastic card. It's not a credit card, just a phone number reference card. I had decided to throw mine away, but knowing that David likes these little cards in his wallet, I thought I would give him his, and so I had put his card on the shelf in the kitchen so I would remember to tell him about it and then he could put it in his wallet. I put mine on the table in the den, in the general direction of the trash. That's where he found the evil little card, the one with my name on it.

He is furious that I got a plastic card with my name on it.

I am furious with him. *Didn't I take the time to think about this? To think that David likes these little cards and he would like to have one of these cards? To set the card aside to give to him instead of immediately dropping it into the trash? Why is it that every time I do something nice for David, it gets thrown back in my face?* I have had it. I actually slap at his arms and tell him I hate him. *I hate him! I hate him!*

The thing is, I really do feel a hateful resentment toward him. I also hate being in this position of trying to do it all, doing things to help him, only to have him turn on me, constantly making an enemy out of me. I have to find a shelf to sit myself on and rise above this. I don't want to hate my own husband. How can I become a better person?

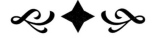

If I could just keep my own emotions out of it. If I could just stop reacting when he pushes my buttons. I practiced trying not to react tonight. So many times. I think I did okay, but then I can't really relax. Instead, I have to connive my way through the night. Outguess and second-guess, role-play and act, but I can never just be myself.

Tonight, David came to me with a look of complete anger on his face. He had the small coffee scoop in his hand. I asked him what was wrong. He said that the big coffee scoop was gone.

"It's GONE!" he exclaimed.

I said, "And you're blaming me? I didn't take your coffee scoop."

"No, I'm not blaming you. I *know* who did it." He then glared over at our grandson, now all of eight years old.

I told David that was ridiculous, but this is where my anger starts to take over. He will keep on and keep on with some crazy notion like this one. Why would Devon have the slightest interest in a coffee scoop? Well, of course, Devon would not have any interest in it, and he would not have touched it. But there is David repeating over and over that he puts it "IN ONE PLACE AND ONE PLACE ONLY" and it is "GONE." "GONE!" Didn't I know how critical it was for him to know that his things are in their places? Didn't I know that when people mess with his stuff, they are messing with his brain?

Actually, I thought this was pretty observant of David and a moment definitely worth savoring. But the moment couldn't be sustained. It lasted only a microsecond and I was immediately back to "Of course, Devon was not the one to move the damn coffee scoop." Move it? That would never happen, because of course, Devon does not care about a stupid coffee scoop!

David goes on to lecture me as to how careful he is. He is always the most careful person about where he puts things.

"No," he tells me. "You are wrong about this. I am right." And he repeats again, "I know exactly who has taken it!"

Again, he is glaring at our grandson and I am trying to get in front of his line of vision so that Devon does not pick up on the fact that he has been so directly targeted.

I direct Devon to the den to watch TV for a few minutes while I go to the kitchen and start to go through all of the cabinets and drawers. Where is the scoop? It's really not there. Where did it go? I noticed that the coffee can was pretty full, so David must have opened a new can. What would he do when opening a new can? *Ah ha! Maybe the scoop is inside the old can and where would the old can be? In the trash.* I invited David to come with me to look just in case there was any possibility of him learning some sort of lesson should the damn scoop be there. And, "Ah ha," there it is at the bottom of the trash can!

David wonders who put it in there, of course.

I can't even talk to him. I pull the coffee scoop out of the trash and hand it to David then go to talk to Devon. I tell Devon that sometimes with Papa's illness, he thinks things have happened that have not actually happened and sometimes he thinks that other people have moved things around. "Sometimes we have to stop what we are doing and help him out." Devon says, "I know." He does know and he won't react now. He will react later.

✦ ✦ ✦ ✦ ✦ ✦

Today, David got angry because I had asked him to shovel some heavy wet spring snow away from the side of the house where we are installing a new door tomorrow. When I got home from work, he was quite upset that no one had showed up to do the work. I told him, as I had previously told him, that Dennis would be installing the door *tomorrow*, first thing in the morning.

I thought that David was angry because he was asked to do the shoveling, but instead, he was angry that he was asked to do the shoveling a full day before the work was to be done.

"What if the wind blows it all back? Then I'll have to do it all over again."

No, I explain that the wind cannot blow the snow because the snow has been on the ground for two weeks now and it is very heavy. It's mid-spring. "The snow can't blow around anymore."

David repeats again that he is worried that the snow is going to blow back. I again try to explain that it cannot blow back.

Every time I come into the kitchen, David is waiting for me so he can continue to question me in an accusatory way as to why

I asked him to shovel snow. I leave the kitchen to avoid a fight. He comes in the den and once again repeats that he should not have been told to shovel snow when the work wasn't being done right away and the snow will all blow back again. Without emotion, I again describe to him the physical characteristics of heavy snow and how the wind cannot move heavy wet snow. This time, he accepts it. Why, I have no idea. Tomorrow, we may be right back to why did I tell him to shovel snow when the wind will just blow it all back, but somehow I reached him tonight. I just wish I knew how I did that.

✦ ✦ ✦ ✦ ✦ ✦

It is becoming absurd—the things that David covets as his own, things that are not to be touched or used by anyone else. He has his own toilet paper and his own spray cleaners. He hides feather dusters in his night stand. Not that he ever uses them anymore, but he had a thing about cleaning and organizing. It was something he thought he was good at, and in fact, he used to be good at it. He was very dedicated to getting the job done, no matter how long it took. That dedication has been missing for a very long time now. Now, it's just about the ownership. How can I convince him that I don't care about feather dusters?

I needed a place where I could feed the cats that was away from the dog, specifically David's dog, the one with the sick stomach. The old wooden desk in the basement seemed to me to be a perfect place. The dogs didn't go in the basement. It was up off the floor so it wouldn't attract ants. David didn't use the desk. But no, David did not want me to set the cat food anywhere near the workshop area of the basement. He said that he needed that space for his work. I asked him what work? I guess that was mean, but it is so obvious that he does no work in the workshop. Isn't it more important to save the dog's life? The dog gets deathly ill from eating anything but dog casseroles that I have to construct out of special grumblies, rice and drained hamburger. Does he have any sympathy for me or the dog? The answer is "No. It's my work area. You are not going to touch my work area. What do you mean there's something wrong with the dog? That dog is fine." So, I guess the cats can eat on top of the dryer for now.

It's yet another problem for me to sort out. Not such a big problem, but on the other hand, I now have dog food and cat food, both dry food and cans, in my closet, in the linen closet, in the coat closet—all to save the dog from being fed or overfed by David during the day when I am at work. Keeping the cat food away from the dog was just one more thing I was trying to do. David knows his dog is sick. He was with me at the vet when I wrote out a check for over $300 to pay for the vet detective work to find out that his dog has mini-bowels in her midsection and requires ultra special care.

I talk to myself like this as though it might make a difference. David might just revert to someone who has a memory, someone who is a responsible and caring adult, and then I can become a nice person again. In reality, I know that what I really have to do is to find another home for David's dog. I know I will never hear the end of this from David, but some things, every once in a while, become clear to me.

I guess I'm a slow learner.

✦ ✦ ✦ ✦ ✦ ✦

Despite all of the negativism, the accusing, the fighting, David's possessiveness and the anger that we both share daily, if not hourly this year, we are happy in our new house. It fits us well, giving David private space in the bedroom or downstairs in the workshop, giving me private space in the den or spare bedroom. These are places that we can run away to when necessary, when we just can't stand each other for a minute more.

We love our back porch. Now that it's April, I am starting to clean it up and plan a Cape Cod decorating scheme out there. Whimsical. Fun. It's nice to think about something positive for a change. The cats, particularly, think they are in heaven as they watch the birds from protected vantage points just inside the screens.

David loves walking the dogs around the block, talking to the neighbors. While I sorely miss the old house my family owned for over 40 years, I can't feel bad about this change. There are no maintenance nightmares in this house. It is not sitting on a busy road with traffic back and forth to the local harbor making David afraid and anxious. No, this was a good decision, a comfort to both of us. In some ways, or maybe in many ways, living in this house makes me think that we are role-playing living out our retirement years before we actually retire.

In reality, we are living out retirement years that we will never have together.

But I can't go there. I just can't go there.

✦ ✦ ✦ ✦ ✦ ✦

So many of our "outings" seem to be for doctor's appointments or lab work, and now we've added dental appointments. Somehow, I forgot that David had not been to a dentist for a long time and I was now the one responsible for him. He needed several appointments for fillings and he's now on a schedule of four cleanings a year to make up for a lack of due diligence. The dentist and staff are very aware of David's illness. He is treated with good-natured fun, caring and respect, so he's never apprehensive about going to his appointments. The receptionist's sister-in-law also has Early Onset Alzheimer's Disease. We talk often, comparing notes.

While we still share a bed and sleep wrapped together, sometimes David just seems to me to be like a big little kid taking up half the bed. He has a shower, gets on his jammies and climbs into bed. There are no worries for him. Not anymore. He doesn't get his clothes ready for the next day. He doesn't set an alarm clock. There is nothing that he needs to prepare for. He will close his eyes and drift peacefully off to sleep.

When he wakes up the next day, he will not have a schedule to keep. He will not read the morning paper. Except for his adult cup of coffee, he will be like a little kindergarten child on his first day, happy and excited, wide-eyed, but also bewildered. Every single day now is a puzzle that he has to sort through, so he takes it ever so slowly. It is so hard for me to match his new pace at slow speed, while I whirl about getting ready for work, cleaning up, making meals, washing clothes and cleaning up the yard.

He is on slow speed. I am on fast speed. It seems that the only times that our paths cross long enough for us to actually look at each other is during lunch and dinner. So, mealtimes are getting longer and more important. It's just evolving that way.

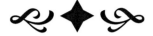

I am finding it a bit harder to remember things that I would like to jot down. I think it is because they have all become so normal to me, so much a normal part of the day that they no longer stand out.

For the past few months, David has been calmer overall. His doctor upped his Paxil to 40 milligrams a day which he now takes at night with his Aricept. It has made all the difference. We haven't had too many of the angry episodes that have so far seemed to characterize this year. Lately, though, after a few months on the higher dose, David is once again becoming periodically angry and difficult to please. That seems to be the way it is with his medication changes. There is an effect, but it is always only temporary. So if it is a good effect, it is only a temporary respite; if it is a bad effect, I have to report it to the doctor and sometimes get David seen again to get his dosages rearranged.

He has had several more falls. Crashes really. I was downstairs in the basement painting when David got up one Saturday, late as usual. I heard him crash to the floor. As I was holding my breath wondering how long to wait before I went upstairs to see if he was okay, there was another distinct crash. He had fallen again. No injuries, but he was upset, very upset at the notion that he could not control what was happening.

I wrote a big note and put it on his bedside table. "DAVID, WHEN YOU GET UP, SIT ON THE BED FOR AT LEAST 30

MINUTES BEFORE YOU GET UP." He has been good about following this instruction. Day after day, he has taken quite a bit of time sitting on the side of the bed to get himself acclimated to a conscious state before moving about the house. No falls.

A few days later, though, I came home to find David very visibly upset with a very large bump and scrape on the top of his head. He had fallen in the bathroom this time, hit and broken the towel rack with his head. Worse, this had occurred later in the day, not when he first got up. Now I was really worried. We had talked to his neurologist about the seizure-like jerks and other falls, but these more serious falls had occurred after our last appointment.

David's neurologist ordered an EEG. The results showed that his responses were slow, but it did not show any seizure activity. When I called the doctor about David's more recent falls, his response was that David needed a walker. He was moving too fast and he needed to stop being so impulsive. He should have the walker for balance and safety. He felt this was a normal progression of the disease.

That diagnosis did not sit well with me at all! David has no balance problems. He has no trouble putting one foot in front of the other and no trouble finding the floor with his feet. Falling like this is more of an advanced-stage symptom of Alzheimer's Disease. I found out from David's sister that she has Meniere's Disease, and it tends to run in families. Meniere's Disease is about losing your balance, dizziness, headaches and falling due to a fluid imbalance in the inner ear. Although David only had the falling symptom, I had found a reference on the Internet to certain Meniere's Disease victims literally "crashing to the floor," with no notice and no aftereffects. At that point, I made an appointment with David's GP. His GP did not think David was having symptoms of Meniere's. Maybe it's TIAs or ministrokes? Maybe it's blood sugar. David's mother was a diabetic. Our next step is to run some fasting blood sugar tests and see what's up. While waiting three weeks for this appointment, David has been fall-free. Was this a phase? Will it happen again?

✦　✦　✦　✦　✦　✦

Yesterday, our grandson was quite busy doing everything possible to antagonize David. He poked him on the butt, did sing-songs of insane word-repeated jingles, and screamed for help with things he could do himself. Basically, he was making everyone pretty miserable, but then, we are adults. We can take it. Enter David, who is a child (as I have to remind myself repeatedly). He could not take it. We were outside. When Devon poked David one too many times, David picked up the shovel I had taken outside to clean up some dirt sludge left by the snow plows. He ran across the lawn with the shovel and chased Devon around the front yard. I ran after David and screamed repeatedly, "Stop!" Finally, he stopped and let me take the shovel from him.

I asked David what he planned to do with the shovel once he caught Devon. He looked at me quizzically and said he had brought the shovel outside to do some shoveling and that was what he planned to do.

"No," I said, trying hard not to burst into tears. "You were chasing our grandson with the shovel, David. What were you going to do if you caught Devon? What on earth were you going to do?"

"Well," David replied calmly, "I was going to shovel."

I turned and put the shovel away in the garage. Incredibly, Devon once again reached over to David to jab him as he walked to the door, and David whipped around, slapping at him with a straight arm and outstretched hand that luckily fell short.

I ushered David into the house, feeling like my heart was thudding to my feet. This is a very dangerous pairing. David can never, never, never be left in any position where he can harm Devon. This is the first time I've clearly seen David being dangerous, and, of all people, to his own grandson! It's hard to take and harder to forget.

About 20 minutes later, I sat Devon down with me in the front yard and we talked about David's brain illness and how Devon is going to have to learn to act older than David. Devon has to act like the parent. I told Devon that I did not blame him for being angry with David, but he could not take out his anger on other people. At the same time, I am realizing how crazy this is. I am telling an eight-year-old child that he has to act like an adult because the adult acts like he is eight years old!

✦ ✦ ✦ ✦ ✦ ✦

It keeps happening.

Devon came to me and told me in an offhand manner that David had kicked him. I said, "No, he didn't really, did he?" Yes, Devon said it again. David had kicked him.

I went to David and said that Devon had told me that he had kicked him. David's response was "Well, he farted on me. He shouldn't do that." I told David that under no circumstances could he kick or hit Devon. Did he understand?

"Sure," David says. I ask him again if he understands.

"Sure," he says again. "But tell him to stay out of my way."

Again, incredibly, after being told to keep a one-foot distance from David, Devon walked up to David and, while keeping a one-foot margin, he farted in David's direction. I grabbed him and put him in a different room where we stayed the rest of the night. I tried to explain to Devon what it meant to provoke David. He said he understood, but what was I expecting? It was unrealistic for the child to control the adult.

Devon then told me that the last time he had come to our house, which was the previous weekend, Devon had brushed up behind David to get a pencil. David shook Devon's head violently with his fists at either side of his head, saying, "Leave me alone," in an angry tone. He then grabbed Devon and threw him to the ground. Devon had not told anyone about this when it happened.

I knew then that my days of having unabashed fun with my grandson were at an end. From now on, his safety had to be first.

I called David's doctor and got a prescription for Xanax to give to David before Devon came over again. I would be glued to Devon's side to prevent any further problems, but at the same time, I knew I was allowing a potentially dangerous situation to occur, just because I wanted to spend time with my grandson. I had a responsibility to watch over David, but I also wanted to spend time with my grandson. I had a responsibility to maintain my grandson's safety. I felt like a rubber band between David and Devon. I prayed that the Xanax would dull David to a nonentity.

✦ ✦ ✦ ✦ ✦ ✦

Yet, it does not get any better. Yes, the Xanax seems to help in that David is not physically responding to Devon, but there is such verbal animosity that it seems just as bad.

When Devon came over this weekend, he had all his ADHD wires charged, and so he jabbered away a million miles an hour. When he walked into the kitchen, he poked at David twice. David whirled around and screamed at Devon to stop. Devon seemed very aloof, but I can tell when he is bothered, and David's reaction certainly bothered him. David then snarled out some comments about what Devon was being allowed to do to him. Devon is allowed to touch him. It was as though he had been sexually harassed. David said that Devon had hit him in the balls.

The thing is, Devon never did that or anything close. As promised, I had stuck to him like glue. I saw him poke a finger at David's arm and poke a finger at David's ribs. It was done in fun. It was the same fun he and his dad had with David, back and forth, on numerous prior occasions. In the old days, everyone would go at it, Dennis, Devon and David, poking and jabbing at each other. Today, though, Devon's poking fun elicited an evil reaction from David. No one in the world could have mistaken his tone for anything but what it was—hatred, pure and simple. He seems to have a world of wrath for Devon, and he is figuring out just how to aim it at him.

I counseled Devon to stay away from David. Remember that David is sick, that his Alzheimer's Disease is making him mean—and that when he is mean, he can be dangerous.

✦ ✦ ✦ ✦ ✦ ✦

We all got in the car to go get some ice cream tonight. Devon aggravated David by pushing at the back of David's seat. I finally had to drive David home and tell him to go in the house. I could not have them both in the car together.

They cannot be in the same car or, for that matter, in the same room together. Lucky that my house has a basement level and perhaps Devon and I can just concentrate ourselves down there, but then how do I supervise David at the same time? This is not feeling very fair. I have to give up my grandson to keep my husband? Part of me wants to tell David that I would much prefer to play with my grandson. Kristin has relied on me to provide her with some relief. Devon has spent a lot of time with me. He's my buddy. I'm not prepared to give that up.

It's unfair, unfair, unfair. It doesn't escape me that I refer to Devon as "my grandson" not "our grandson." David has forever lost his rights to be a grandfather to Devon. Where is the David who loved him so? Where is the David who used to drive Devon around in his truck until he got sleepy? They would go down to the harbor to look at the boats and the water.

Where is Devon's grandfather? Papa is gone forever. I try to explain the situation to Kristin. Devon's visits have become a problem. He just can't come over as often. I am sad. I will try to find a way to spend some time with Devon, but it can't be in the same house with David.

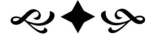

I so much want to capture the moments that still sometimes define us as husband and wife, as a team, as friends, as us against the world. Isn't that what all of us want in a marriage, someone we look forward to coming home to? It's what defines marriages. Having that mate, that partner. Someone you can be absolutely comfortable with. Someone you can tell your secrets to. The old moments that used to define us are so hard to remember. We do have moments, but they are always taking on new shapes and dimensions.

A cup of regular coffee in the middle of the afternoon at Dunkin' Donuts is still an old moment that we can share. We always drink our coffee black, but in the middle of a Saturday or Sunday afternoon, there's nothing better than a cup of steaming creamy sweet coffee that only Dunkin' Donuts seems to know how to make. I drive us to Dunkin' Donuts. I order the coffee and I pay for it, but then we sit down together to enjoy it. It's a ritual.

It used to be a ritual that David would go to the dump on Sundays. Now, we go to the dump together. I collect the bags of garbage from inside and outside, making sure that everything is bagged up. I put the bags in the truck or hand them to David and direct him to put them in the truck. I drive. David unloads the bags into the big dump truck receptacles. That's his job. It takes him a while, but part of the new ritual is that I sit patiently in the truck while he carefully unloads the garbage bags and throws them one by one into the big dump truck receptacles.

Time has no meaning for David. He has one speed — extra slow. It's okay. We are just doing things differently together now.

At least we are still together.

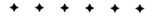

Fifteenth of May, David's 56th birthday. We took a cruise to Bermuda and had a great time! A local travel agency had arranged van transportation to Boston from our local shopping center up the street. It was impossible to get lost and so very easy for me as David's caregiver. The hardest part was packing and thinking ahead for two people. David stayed close by my side and only lost his way once; on the ship, he left dinner to go to the bathroom one night and got disoriented. I had all the ship staff out looking for him that night, but somehow he found his way back to our cabin an hour later.

The natural beauty in Bermuda was phenomenal. We walked, shopped, swam and went snorkeling. More than any other activity, the snorkeling seemed to give David more joy and true independence than I had seen in a long time. He was truly comfortable in the water and as awestruck as I was by the impossibly brilliant colors of the fish and the aqua blue water and sky. No one in our group had any idea that David had an illness.

For the most part, I was able to ignore it as well. We were able to reconnect as a couple, spending time together that was not consumed by having to deal with the daily problems we were getting all too used to at home.

✦ ✦ ✦ ✦ ✦ ✦

Now that we have been back for a few weeks, David is in an agitated phase. I should say, superagitated. It has been going on now for three days. In this phase, he hates me with such a venom and passion it seems to literally seethe out of his mouth in everything he says to me. This is how he was acting with Devon only a few months ago. Now I am the target. Or maybe more truthfully, I am the target once again.

He has a special tone he reserves for me and it is clearly *I hate you. I despise you. I hate you.* Today, he was up at 6:15 in the morning. I have seen this before, his anger and agitation preventing him from sleeping. He will get up early, not really even knowing himself why he is up. Once up, he is into drinking coffee after coffee, which only makes it worse.

He found his keys to the truck and drove himself to Dunkin' Donuts where he bought himself yet another coffee—a giant iced coffee. He has not driven at all for a solid two months. He hates me so much right now that it is taking something really big to show me, like driving when he knows he should not drive. He pretends that his doctor did not tell him to stop driving. He says I made it up to control him, to force him to sit in the house day after day.

It seemed to start with a note I had written on a little sticky paper and put beside the fern in the basement bathroom. It said, "Please don't water me anymore, I'm drowning." An innocuous stupid little note. The poor little plant was totally soaked and sitting in two inches of water. A few days before, I had discovered it similarly soaked along with a fern in David's bathroom.

David screamed at me for assuming that he was the one who had touched the plant. He said he absolutely did not and I was the scoundrel of the universe for thinking it was him. He came to me with this newsflash at least four times over the day, with no conversation in between. When Kristin called, he told me that I had better ask her, because she was the person I should have accused. Why don't I just go ahead and accuse her so he can be cleared of this offense.

"But noooo," he exclaims, "you would never say 'I'm sorry.' Nooo. Not you. You are too high and mighty to apologize, aren't you?"

He was already in this hateful mood when he discovered that I had trimmed some bushes. The bushes were near the bird feeders he fills regularly and David became livid, saying that I had killed the birds with my stupidity. I did it on purpose. I knew that he took care of that area. It was his area and I just went in and ripped it apart. I have now killed all the birds.

I tried to explain to David that the birds sit in the trees, not in the bushes, but it was useless. How could I do it? How? Why didn't I just ask? Why did I have to be so stupid and cruel?

Well, the world is lopsided to such a degree I can't put it right. I did not harm the birds and if I temporarily disoriented them, it was not on purpose. I simply cleaned up the dead bushes and freed up the nice pines that were struggling for room and, god forbid, I planted some flowers. What a crime. I will never live it down!

He sneers at me, coming in to examine my coffee cup to see if I have any coffee left when he has none at the moment. He has, in fact, drained the pot in the kitchen now at least three times today. He is angry that I have not made more coffee.

He snarls at me, "No, you never make any coffee, do you? Not you. Nooo. You're too special, aren't you?"

He walks out the front door and glares at the dandelions in the front yard, standing with arms akimbo for huge dramatic effect, walking slowly, stopping, shaking his head. He comes in and tells me how stupid and pigheaded I am and how I don't know what I'm doing. I cannot do enough lawn treatments to calm his agitation about the dandelions, the dead bushes, the coffeepot and whatever else he needs to address right now to assert some control.

At 11:30 last night, he wanted to know what I have done with all his money. If I don't tell him, he tells me that he will just have to go through everything on my desk. At midnight, he woke me up to ask about the Krugerrands I have invested in. I haven't invested in Krugerrands. I didn't even know what they were, much less how to spell the word until I looked it up to figure out what he was talking about. Now our world is getting very odd indeed.

The laundry that David used to take great pride in is in strange piles, sitting all over the basement. He keeps coming down to fold something or organize something, but it doesn't make any sense. Shirts are jumbled over by the workbench. Towels and socks are mixed in half-folded piles.

I gave David two Xanax yesterday, hoping to make a difference, but it did not seem to have any effect. Today, Kristin came over and got an earful about "your mother." She gave him a Xanax too. It had no effect. He is angry, morose, depressed, scowling. He does not have a nice word to say about anything. Devon tells me I should not be living with him. I tell him "thank you." It's the nicest thing anyone has said to me all day!

I will be glad to leave for work tomorrow.

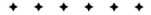

We have had a full seven days of this now with no letup. I am very surprised. I keep expecting that David will flip out of this mood the same way he flipped into it—suddenly. That has not happened.

He accused me of peeing in his toilet and not flushing it. "Webster's," he declares. "Denial. Look it up. You never say you're sorry."

Last night, David told me, "There's a word to describe you. I can't think of the word, but it's people like you." A couple of hours later he said, "Paranoia. Do you know that word?" I thought that was interesting and asked him if he thought *he* was paranoid. His answer was "Absolutely not!"

He has brought up the bird killing at least four or five times in the last few days. It's sad that he thinks the birds have died. Now he has removed the birdfeeders. At least it's June now, so the birds shouldn't miss the feeders. I asked him where they were and he said that he put them in "that room, that room beside the house." The garage? "Yes—they're too much trouble. I'm never going to go through all that trouble again."

He complains routinely about how many clothes I have and how he has nothing. Yet at least eight shirts hang ironed and ready in his closet, and four pairs of pants, a few pairs of jeans, eight or nine T-shirts of various colors are all ready to wear. He has three jackets, five baseball caps. He has never been interested in clothes, but he is not without clothes because I now provide and launder and iron all of his clothes and I do a great job. I'm defensive about it because I have put a lot of effort into it. When I come home from work, I find my closet doors open. I think he is counting my clothes.

I found one of the newest baseball caps I bought for David in the garbage last night. I asked why he threw it away—it cost $15. He said because it was not a Red Sox cap. It may have looked like a Red Sox cap, but it said *Indians* on the back so he didn't like it for that reason. Yet the previous week, he wore it all the time and told me several times how much he loved it.

He questions why I close the drapes at night and pull down the blinds.

"Why do you always do that? What is wrong with you that you do that?"

I explain the appropriateness. He wants to know where it is written that I should do that. He wants to see out. He does not agree that if I open the blinds at night anyone can see in. He does not consider it a problem at all. Whenever he walks through the living room or when he is in the kitchen at night, he pulls on the cords drawing open the drapes or blinds. I ask him not to do it, explaining that it is 7:00 at night. He says, "No, it's not. It's daytime."

Last night, I had to attend a board meeting and was careful to tell David that I had to go out, when I would be back, and that I would make dinner as soon as I got back. Kris called me on my cell phone an hour and a half later. She had just seen David driving down a street in her neighborhood. She came over to the house to find David back at the house and very agitated. He came out of the house throwing his arms up in the air saying loudly, "Where is everybody?"

Kristin said that for a minute she felt like she was eight years old again and dealing with her drunken dad, with everyone running all around trying to get out of his way. It seemed much the same to me as well. David's aggression toward me has been exactly like what it was like when he was drinking heavily.

This is not good, because I made a commitment to myself that I would never again allow myself to be subjected to this treatment. Yet here I am again. How am I supposed to deal with this?

Kris made us both dinner and gave her dad another Xanax. She went beyond that and called his doctor the next day, relating to him exactly what was going on. In her view, David's aggression toward me comes just short of using physical force. It is verbal abuse. Will David be able to control himself? His doctor said that it sounded like David needs a little sedation. He refilled the Xanax and started him on Risperdal twice a day.

When I came home from work tonight, I found David sleeping. He woke up but would hardly look at me. This week, every time I ask David how he is doing his answer is "What does it matter?" or "What do you think?" If I remark on the weather or say something to the dogs, there is no spark of conversation. He does not want to talk to me.

Later, I started to ask him if he wanted to go to the store with me but he interrupted me with a loud and forceful "No." I started laughing, thinking he was joking around, but he was serious. I got as far as "Would you like to…" "NO!" I suggested that he might want to get out. We could go have dinner, pick up his prescriptions and go to the store. He finally very reluctantly agreed.

He sat in the back seat of the car. Why? "So I won't get hurt."

He groaned and growled because he could not pull out the seat belt. I stopped the car. He got out in a huff to pull off the sweatshirt that was making him hot. I fixed the seat belt. He got back in but would not put the seat belt on. I felt like I was driving around a six-year-old child.

When we arrived, he stood outside the car, trying four times over to get his sweatshirt back on the right way, stamping his feet. He was obviously irritated. He started talking about all the cars in the parking lot.

We went out to dinner where he talked nonstop about all the cars and how bad they were and how they have ruined the environment. He said that people who used to ride bicycles had it right when they did not have cars back then. A picture hung on the wall showing two ladies from the early 1900s standing beside two bicycles. He said over and over how much he loved the picture and wanted to have it.

Back in the car, he started talking about the birds again, but he said that it didn't matter now that they were dead and he wasn't going to feed them anymore.

Kris called while we were putting away groceries in the kitchen. When I returned to the kitchen, David was glaring. He said that he was pissed about the milk, the "one-percent milk." He said he was very pissed. "That silly stuff. You're throwing away all the good stuff by getting that." I explained that it is only lower fat, not lower calcium. "Why do you do that? What good is it to do that? You are just throwing it away. For what? You should be out walking and riding a bike like I do. But you never do that."

I found the lettuce in the freezer. I told David that lettuce cannot go into the freezer. He replied that of course lettuce can go in the freezer. He explained that he put it in there while sorting stuff out, while organizing the groceries. He knew it was there. "It's okay if you know it's there." He likes his lettuce cold, and, besides, I was blocking the refrigerator. I had been blocking the refrigerator all night. He told me that I am his worst enemy and followed it with "Did you hear what I said? You are my worst enemy."

He wanted to start a fight, but I went to bed. He went into his bathroom and brought out an empty box of tissues. What did I have to say about that? I told him that I did not know what he was talking about.

He held up the box and said, "This—don't tell me you don't know. You know. Of course, you know. It was half a box and now there are none. See? It's empty."

I said, "So you think I took your tissues? Is that it?"

"It was half a box and now it's empty," he replies in an accusatory tone. It's now 11:00 p.m. I am tired. So tired. Over and over. He's like a broken record. He told me that I was not getting it. I repeated that I had not touched his box of tissues.

"You take care of yourself, don't you? You take all the good stuff for yourself. You make sure that you're well taken care of, don't you?" I pull the covers over my head. Even if I don't respond, he won't stop. He just keeps badgering me. I don't know how to deal with this. I keep waiting for it to stop. It seems to be all about what I have that he does not have. He views me as conceited, self-obsessed, self-indulgent, controlling, and, oh yes, cruel. I told him tonight that he is going to have to get used to the fact that I am his caregiver and that I have to make the decisions. He laughed derisively and asked what do I do to take care of him.

✦ ✦ ✦ ✦ ✦ ✦

Add depression to my endearing qualities now. It's 8:15 in the morning and I was due at work 15 minutes ago. I have no desire to do a thing. I don't want to be badgered any more. I have no makeup or shoes on and I haven't done my hair. I'm getting tired of trying to take care of David and everything else. I can live with being unappreciated, but I cannot live with this constant badgering. I will be giving him a Xanax as soon as I get home tonight. Maybe we can get a jump-start on his mood before it becomes really bad tonight.

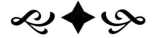

It's now mid-June. David continues to have the nighttime body jerking while he sleeps. These are frequent but relatively minor body jerks. It's becoming more routine now that he is also having significant body jerking during the day, the kind that seems to shock his whole body. That's when whatever is in his hands goes flying. I seem to be constantly cleaning up flying coffee from the table and the floor. Sometimes it's days before I notice that drips of coffee have ended up on the walls and even the ceiling. We've had a few flying lunches as well. Tomato soup. Salami sandwiches. I laugh. David laughs too but then he also apologizes. I tell him it's all right. It doesn't matter and I run to replace whatever it is.

I'd like to believe that the falls that David has had so far are just the result of periodic ultra-extreme body jerks, but I just don't know. He fell twice on Saturday, but out of my view. This is getting worrisome. I need to see him fall to know what is going on.

The next day, my wish comes true and it all becomes very clear. I was sitting on the porch, reading the Sunday paper. David was sleeping late as usual, but then he got up by himself and started to walk from the bedroom, down the hall, across the dining room toward the kitchen. From the corner of my eye, I could see him striding purposefully toward the kitchen. Then suddenly, he was no longer moving forward, he was crashing downward. There was no body jerking at all. He simply crashed to the floor.

It was a weird sort of slow motion, as I turned my head to fully look in his direction. By then, he had disappeared behind the dining room table. Then just as quickly, he emerged, rising up again, almost returning to a full standing position when again, he crashed to the floor. It was surreal. How could this be? My husband is so physically healthy. He is anything but frail. In fact, he's the opposite of frail. He's sturdy, muscular, strong. So how could he be in a heap on the floor? In disbelief, I ran to him and started to pull him up, telling him we had to get him back to the bed.

I held onto him as best I could, and as we were walking toward the bedroom, down he went again, face first with his arms straight down and extended rigidly behind him. He was very unfocused and unable to respond clearly to me.

Somehow I pulled and dragged him to the bed. I had to yell and push and pull him down to get him to sit and then to lie back in the bed. Then I ran and grabbed the video camera. One of my greatest frustrations over the past several months had been not being able to adequately describe to David's neurologist what these extreme body jerks and drops were like. I was determined to get David on tape. In fact, this time I finally got quite a bit on tape with David lying on the bed in his unfocused state, exhibiting multiple extreme body jerks with his arms shooting out straight even as he lay prone in the bed.

It was about 20 minutes later when David complained that he really had to get up to go to the bathroom. I tried to hold him back, but he said he really had to go. As soon as he got into the bathroom, he fell again. I was prepared. I had wrapped my arms around him and so he sank against me. He managed to go to the bathroom and then I ushered him back into bed.

Another 30 minutes went by. David's condition slowly improved. When I videotaped him again, he was much more focused but continued to have these seizure-like jerking movements.

We were both very distressed by this course of events. While he was jerking, I was shaking. It was scary for both of us. Of course, I called his doctor and was told to take David to the emergency room. By then, the episode was over. The ER doctor felt that the culprit was the Risperdal that had been added to David's medications the week before to tone down his aggression. Apparently it was too much for him, as it can lower the threshold for seizure activity. I was told to add Risperdal to the list of medications that David should never take again. It's too dangerous for him and too dangerous for me.

So, does this mean that I must return to the verbal abuse from David that I had to experience before the Risperdal? As we leave the hospital, I am feeling doomed to this odd balancing act that we now live day to day. Try one thing. Try something else. Try to survive the days in between. We can try to minimize the seizures, but without additional meds on board, we'll be back to David's constant badgering, accusations and bad mood. The seizures scared me. The aggression wears me out. There is simply no good answer.

The video I took, though, turned out to be a godsend. David's neurologist was clearly quite impressed and said that these seemed to be frontal seizures, of which there is no standard pattern. He started David on Depakote three times a day. He felt that it would help David's mood as well. I was willing to try it. As with everything else, we will just wait and see.

So, we are in a new reality now. One step forward. Two steps back. More meds. What's next?

✦ ✦ ✦ ✦ ✦ ✦

Part of the new reality is accepting that I can no longer leave David entirely alone for so many hours a week. I absolutely know that I'm taking a chance each and every morning when I pull out of the driveway to go to work. It's starting to weigh heavily on me and certainly adding to my stress. I am leaving one job for another. Will David stay in bed for most of the day? Will he answer my phone calls from work to let me know that he is all right? He has already said that he does not want anyone else in the house. We haven't talked about it at length, but we have talked about it. "That is not going to happen," he told me quite firmly. "Just forget about that idea."

Yet in our support group, we talk quite a bit about the need to rely on others, to have someone come into our homes to help provide supervision and, much more importantly, to provide some much-needed caregiver respite for ourselves. Not that it's a comfortable thought for me either, the idea of having someone in our house whom we do not know. It does seem like a major invasion of privacy, and in an odd and maybe stupid way, it also feels like we are giving in to illness rather than fighting against it.

So, what now? We had already lost David's income. We just couldn't lose mine too.

I was the director of human resources for a nonprofit agency providing services to children and families. While I was feeling quite overwhelmed by all of this, feeling lodged between a rock and a hard place, my assistant tendered her resignation. *Great*, I thought, *now I will have to do her job in benefits administration plus my job until I can fill the position. This is just what I needed*. Then an idea slowly came to me. *What if I just did her job?* Her job has boundaries. Mine does not. Her job can be run independently from any location. Mine requires that I be present among the managers at our central administrative headquarters. What if I demoted myself and ran her job mostly from my home? I could be there for David. I could be home.

My agency and our CEO were incredibly supportive. It took a few months, but they hired a new director of human resources and allowed me to take over the benefits work. Now, I go in to the main office twice a week in the mornings. The rest of the time, I work from home. My day now starts at 5:00 a.m., so I can get an early start in my home office, which is in the study in our basement. While David sleeps until noon, I do most of my work for the day. Then I take a two-hour break to help David get up, to fix lunch and take the time to sit down and eat with him. In the late afternoon, I finish my workday down in the basement, while David sits in the den upstairs or walks around holding the little dog. He patiently waits for me to return to start dinner.

There is no mistaking David's reaction to this new arrangement. He is comfortable and secure. There is less agitation. There is less anger. How much of the anger of this past year has really been about his insecurity?

✦　✦　✦　✦　✦　✦

We are surrounded by the colors of fall. It's now mid-October, and I am well immersed into my new work and home schedule. I go in to the main office on Monday and Friday mornings. It's good to work from home. David says he likes my being here. I'm fixing nutritional lunches and we are spending more time together. David gets on the elliptical machine once or twice a day. We are both walking. Things are better.

I found a wonderful home for David's dog, Annie. In addition to her digestive problems, Annie had also started cowering in the closet each time David had any seizure activity. All it would take was a jerk of the arm or a coffee cup flying up in the air, and off she would go to the closet, refusing to come out, even when David called for her. He had always been so sweet to her. What a sad thing to be rejected by your own dog because of your illness. David, quite surprisingly, had no reaction at all to Annie secreting herself in the closet or refusing to come to him. He also had no reaction to giving her away. The day she left, I thought it would be so traumatic for him. He waved good-bye and that was it. Oddly enough, he still refers to the dogs in plural. He has to let the dogs in or let the dogs out or take the dogs for a walk. He will walk around for hours with the little dog. He never looks for Annie and never asks about her.

I'm glad to have simplified our lives, but as for me, Annie's loss does hurt.

✦　✦　✦　✦　✦　✦

David is now into delusional thinking. He has brought a long-term memory forward to fill a short-term memory space. He accused me of throwing away his bike, the one he tells me he has been riding all around…his beautiful, perfect, fantastic bike. In fact, he was talking about the racing bike he had in Hawaii, not a bike from last month or last year. It was 29 years ago that we left Hawaii, and I don't know what happened to that bike. David probably gave it away to someone he liked along the way. That's his personality. If someone he met liked something that he had, he would give it to him or her. We have moved so many times. He has given away so much over the years. Where is the bike? What happened to it? I have no idea. I only know that we have not owned that bike for nearly 30 years.

I hadn't thought about those days in Hawaii for such a long time. David was so tan, strong and lanky back then in his bike-racing days. He loved it, riding 20 miles a day to prepare for 100-milers. I would spend an entire Saturday at the epicenter of the race, watching his times. He had a feather-light bike, all the racing gear and gloves, even a training track that we kept in the living room. That was a time when he was athletic and goal-driven. After we left Hawaii and after both of our children were born, David was much more into intellectual thought, philosophy and government, local and national politics. He sailed and walked, but he never rode a racing bike again. Maybe it was just the all-too-perfect weather in Hawaii that inspired him to be so sports-oriented. Once we got back to the mainland, we had not only the seasons to contend with, but jobs in busy metropolitan areas as well. Gone was the peaceful expanse of beach roads begging for daily cycling enthusiasts.

Consumed by this delusional thinking now, David is very aggressively angry toward me. He gets right in my face, accusing me of the theft of his bike. I thought the memory would pass, but it has not. He grabs on to this thought every day. He talks about his beautiful bike, shakes his head and looks at me in a disgusted manner.

Next, he accuses me of stealing his CDs. He is convinced that I either stole them or threw them out. If possible, he is even angrier about this. I tried to explain that I do not touch his CDs. While I can appreciate the music he so loves—Steely Dan, Van Morrison, Dire Straits—it's not my first choice in music. I would much rather listen to something classical. So, I never so much as borrow his CDs. I can appreciate how important they are to him. I understand that it's not just about the music, it's about the possession, the ownership. He regularly sorts and hides them in different places. I regularly go through the house, pick them up and carefully return them to his dresser or to the CD shelves in the den, but now several of the disks are missing from their cases. What has he done with the disks? I start to hide the empty cases so he won't think that I've stolen the CDs out of the cases. It doesn't matter what I do. He is convinced that I am the CD thief.

✦ ✦ ✦ ✦ ✦ ✦

I am slow to realize sometimes that David is building up resentments, which he harbors until they explode from him in angry and accusatory outbursts. I may be totally unaware that this is happening. Last night, after taking him to a wonderful movie, we had just arrived home. He was attaching the lead to the little dog's collar and was having trouble doing it. He refused my help. Suddenly he blurted out how uncaring, unsupportive, mean and ignorant I am that I did not stop at Dunkin' Donuts on the way back from the movie. I explained that Dunkin' Donuts was not on our way back, but in another direction. He continued on about how self-absorbed I am, about how he never gets out of "this fucking hellhole," about how I only care about myself.

Not 10 minutes later, he became incensed over a sheet of white ruled paper that I had placed on the counter to write out the grocery list. He accused me of stealing his paper and using it up. Of course, it didn't matter that it wasn't his paper, and in any case, it wasn't being used up, but I knew not to go there. It would have been a wasted effort. He told me I used to be a nice person, I used to have ethics, but now I am a very bad person. He doesn't know me anymore because of how bad I am.

This, of course, ruined a very nice evening that we had had out of the house. It would be easier to disengage from society, to lock ourselves away. Trying to do the things we used to do just ends up being not worth the effort.

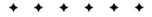

At our last support group meeting, we had new members. A woman in maybe her early 50s with Alzheimer's Disease and her husband, who seemed quite educated and knowledgeable about a variety of related topics. His mother had Alzheimer's Disease and, as a veteran, was treated by the VA. In fact, his mother had been admitted to a VA long-term-care unit where she received superior care. Another member of our group was already taking advantage of his VA benefits and was being seen periodically at a VA hospital a couple of hours away. His wife indicated that he had already been accepted for future long-term care at this facility.

David was a 20-year career veteran. He had 10 years' service in the Navy and 10 years' service in the Coast Guard. Yet when I had checked with the VA, I was told multiple times and without equivocation that there would be no VA long-term care for David, unless he was determined to have a 70 percent service-connected disability. In other words, his disability had to have arisen from or during his career while he served in the Navy or Coast Guard. And just to make it even clearer for me, I was told that Alzheimer's Disease would never be considered an acceptable disability related to his military service.

The other thing that I was told was that the list to get VA medical care is extremely long. You must become enrolled in the VA, and that does not happen automatically. There is a priority list, and while I am welcome to enroll David, he most certainly will not be high on the priority list. Even soldiers coming back from Iraq are finding it difficult to qualify for VA care. I was incensed at that. It was bad enough that David may not be able to get VA medical care, but returning soldiers from Iraq?

I wondered what I was doing wrong to get this response, while it seemed that others were apparently getting a different response. I also wondered if David may be missing out on some excellent state-of-the-art care that he should be getting if he qualified under the VA. As far as immediate medical care, so far I had not been that concerned. We had a military variation of medical insurance through Tufts. Of course, Tufts would not be providing any long-term care for David.

The thought of having to plan for long-term care was distant in my mind. I had too many immediate concerns to worry about. It was enough for me to think that maybe I could do it myself with David remaining in his own home, our home. If it turned out to be too much for me, well then I could have an assistant move in with us. Finally, if that didn't work, we would just have to divest ourselves of our diminishing assets and file for Medicaid. That was my plan, or perhaps my lack of planning. I didn't want to have to think about anything else.

Well, I now have the VA enrollment packet to fill out and I feel compelled to fully explore every avenue, so I promise myself that I will get to it sometime soon. Yet I am feeling so inadequate. In my now palpable stress, I am becoming intolerant of people who try to help. The more resources I have to check out further, the more stressed I become. These are people trying to help me, and all they do is make me angry.

✦ ✦ ✦ ✦ ✦ ✦

Through our support group, I also found out about a day program that David can join. One of our support group members participates in it. It's two towns away, but I made a few calls, and the town next door has a senior services van that will come to pick David up. I found the cost for the program prohibitive and wondered how a program for an adult can cost so much more than a day-care program for a child. It didn't seem to make sense. Still, I signed David up for two days a week. Doing my job at home with David needing more attention was already starting to get difficult. This would give me a chance to focus.

On a beautiful October day, we went together to visit the center. It was modern and inviting. David really liked the artwork displayed on the walls. He has become so visual, instantly attracted to photographs, art, colors and clouds in the sky. He was immediately comfortable and laughed and joked with the providers and participants. I noticed that the participants were quite elderly. David didn't seem to notice at all. He talked and smiled. They talked and smiled. It all seemed so right.

The first day the van came to pick David up, I thought my heart would break into two pieces, right on the front steps of our house. I helped David into his jacket. We talked to the van driver awhile. David kept right on smiling and talking and then he climbed aboard and the driver fastened his seat belt for him. I waved to him as the van pulled away and he waved back.

When I stepped back into the house, I realized that it was the first time that I had been alone in our house since we had moved in. I couldn't believe that my husband was riding around in a Council on Aging van. There was a lady already on the van sharing the ride with David. She looked to be about 85. My husband is only 56 years old. How do I make sense of this picture?

✦ ✦ ✦ ✦ ✦ ✦

I am astounded by the ruination of our lives via this disease and our inability to deal with it in a rational and practical manner. Anyone reading this would think that we are both horrible people, and all we do is mete out blows to each other's psyches. They would forgive David, because he is ill. They would not forgive me! I know that I appear to be frustrated, impatient and angry all the time, and I know that my lack of confidence as a caregiver is all too apparent. I try hard to be the supportive, caring and totally devoted partner to meet David's growing needs for care. I do not write much about so sadly missing the person I married, but I do miss him with all of my heart. We are still trying to live a lifetime together, or what should be a lifetime. Neither one of us is willing to give in to or even talk about the possibility that this lifetime together is limited.

What seemed to be getting better, or working better, was only temporary. It's now the end of the year. Snowy cold, blustery weather has turned us inward, and so we pass the days in our protective igloo.

Although David is putting on weight, probably from the seizure meds, he is quite captivated about his looks. He is convinced that he is sleek, thin and very handsome and will look at himself in the mirror often. He remarks about his physique and his good looks every day. For a few months, he got on the elliptical machine at least once a day. It became one of his compulsive behaviors. So much so, that I had to watch out for him and get him off the machine after 30 minutes. The elliptical machine did not seem to be able to keep up with his weight gain. He has a belly he never had before. His cheeks are puffy and he looks pale to me. Now he has stopped exercising altogether.

He sleeps even more now, up to 16 hours straight, on a regular basis if I don't wake him up. On the days when he goes to the Senior Center, I have to rouse him up at least two hours before, just to get him slowly acclimated to being awake again. Most days, he will not walk the dog or even take the dog outside unless I ask him to. By the time he puts on coat, hat and gloves, he has forgotten what he was going to do. Some days, he just wears his jammies or sweat pants all day and wanders around the kitchen, moving objects from counter to counter.

I am astounded by the changes in David over this past year. Why did I ever think that this disease is progressing slowly? That thought has been on my mind a lot lately, but I don't know what put it there. Is it possible that David was driving only seven or eight months ago? Is it possible that he actually purchased food at a grocery store within the last year? How did he ever carry on these long arguments with me? Now, it would be an impossibility. About half the time now, David cannot complete a sentence. He has started to lose his verbal abilities.

Sentences just start and end in mid-air. Today in the car, he was looking out the window and said, "Oh, look, they have put in new..." I waited, but there was only air. By the time I asked, "New what?" he had forgotten what he was commenting about.

He is so totally dependent on me now. From finding the neck hole in his sweater to warming up a cup of coffee, to turning on the TV for him, to telling him to brush his teeth, to turning the sock on his foot around so that the heel is in the right place, to putting sugar on his cereal or cutting up his food.

I am also astounded at his many episodes of anger and aggressiveness. As we edge toward the new year, there have been several more days of extreme anger and rejection of me as a partner and caregiver. Again, somehow in my mind, I think that *now* is the most terrible time, not before. Before, it was easy. It's the now that's difficult. Well, taken in perspective, it looks like the whole year was difficult and *now* is just more of the same.

More than anything, this year has demonstrated that David seems to be screaming out, "I won't go down without a fight!" Indeed, his past ability to compromise and cover up what was happening has clearly turned into a refusal to accept reality. I am worried about him rejecting me as his caregiver more frequently or to a greater degree. I'm worried about him becoming physically aggressive as he increasingly cannot control his anger and frustration. I'm worried about my ability to weather his moods and personality changes.

Year Five

Most days, David spends time in our bedroom. Sometimes he doesn't appear to be doing anything at all but sitting, ruminating. Other times, he is rearranging his closet or dresser drawers. Sleeping more during the day. Sometimes lying back down on the bed after being up only a few hours.

What I worry about is that he is now closing the door. If I try to open it, he will slam it shut. While he does not appear angry, he acts angry. He hates my role as caregiver and he hates me for being his caregiver. Why can't I just leave him alone, he demands to know.

A few times he has managed to lock the door, after throwing out some of my things. I get panicked with that, wondering what trouble he could be getting into in there.

He told me that he was going to trim some trees in the back yard but couldn't find the chainsaw. Where did I hide the chainsaw? While the hackles went up on the back of my neck, I told him that I didn't think it was a good idea right now and that it's something we should do together in the spring. David scowled at me and stamped his way down to the bedroom complaining about me hiding all his things. I immediately went into the garage, pulled the chainsaw out and hid it.

I am also seeing some very different and difficult mood and behavior swings. Sometimes now, David will take a childlike stance. He will have a little grin on his face and talk to me like I am the parent. "Please, please can I have some ice cream?" At first, I thought he was being sarcastic, but then I realized it was for real. He gallops around the room and leaps on the bed, laughing. If I give him something to eat that he really likes, he will smack his lips saying, "Yum, yum, goody, goody."

He especially likes our little dog and will hold him in his lap or walk around the house with him. I'm thankful for that. They are good for each other. But then, he also walks around the house sometimes holding a doll. It's a funny little stuffed man doll with a pull string in the back. When you pull the string, the man doll says things like "Sure, honey. I'll rub your back. And is there anything else I can get for you?" It's a doll full of comedy routines that used to send our whole family into stitches laughing. Now, it's a comfort doll for an adult who no longer thinks or acts like an adult.

I am dressing David when he needs help, which has now become most of the time. It started slowly. I was purposefully inconspicuous so as not to embarrass him. I would tug here and pull there. It helped him if I laid his clothes out on the bed. Then it grew to helping him put arms in sleeves, head in neck of sweater, zip jacket or pants, put belt in belt holes or tighten the belt. David can occasionally still get dressed, but it can take him up to an hour and a half and he will put on whatever is in front of him. He does not fight me about this area of caregiving. I find that odd, but he seems to like my taking this time with him. I think it is the time together that is most important to him.

When I lay out his clothes, sometimes David ignores them and pulls out his own clothes to put on. It's not a problem unless it's one of his days to go to the Senior Center. On those days, I always have him dressed casually but smartly in color-coordinated cords, plaid shirt and pullover sweater with matching socks and boat shoes or cool sneakers. It's the female version of how to dress a man, but I am convinced that he never did this job as well as I have been doing it for him. It gives me some small measure of satisfaction.

The hardest part has been that David continues to steadily gain weight due to his medications and lack of exercise. I have already packed up and put away the size 34 waist and size 36 waist pants and medium shirts. He now needs size XL (extra large) in almost everything. I will get a whole outfit ironed and put together and then struggle to help David into it, only to find out that it no longer fits.

When I pull a sweater over David's head and guide his arms into the sleeves, he says, "Owie...owie!" Am I hurting him? I don't know. He doesn't know. I ask him and he says, "Yes," then he says, "No." Is it just the discomfort of having someone else dress you? Is it just the weird embarrassment of it all that he is reacting to?

I am also starting to help David with his grooming, putting out what he will need on the counter right beside the sink. I lay out his toothbrush and toothpaste, his shaving cream and razor. I distract him with laughter or news about the weather, anything. I just keep talking as I reach out to fix what he misses or fill in what he can't figure out to do next. I keep pulling out the electric razor for him to use and, occasionally, I find him in the bathroom in the middle of the afternoon, pulling it over his face.

On some of the afternoons when David sits behind a closed door in the bedroom, he is trying in vain to pull his feet through an undershirt. Once he came into the kitchen with an entire leg through the head hole of an undershirt and had it bunched up at his waist, just fine with it. He was wearing another T-shirt on his upper half, backwards, but with head and arms in the right place. I think this success must have taken him two hours. I say something like "Wouldn't you be more comfortable if we find your jeans?"

✦ ✦ ✦ ✦ ✦ ✦

A few months after David started attending the Senior Center, he came home one day shaking his head in disgust, saying, "That asshole. He hit me. Right here." And he pointed to his head. "How could they let him do that?" he asked in a very disgusted tone.

I looked at David's head and ran my fingers through his hair. I could see no mark or scrape nor any evidence that he had been hurt in any way. Still, David was pulling his head away, saying, "Ow. It hurts."

He was convinced that his friend at the Senior Center, our friend who was in our support group, had cuffed him on the side of the head and had done so while sitting right next to the attendant. Of course, I called to find out what had happened. There was no way, said the attendant, that David could have been hit by his friend. David's friend pushed him at one point, a gentle push to the shoulder, but that was all. Maybe it was over dessert. But there were no loud words, no altercation, no fight, and certainly no hitting. The attendant was sitting at the same table.

So I was left to figure out if this was true. Did it really happen? Did David make it up? Or worse, was he getting so paranoid that he really thought that a gentle push to the shoulder was a blow to the head? Or, perhaps even worse than that, was this delusional thinking entirely made up in his own mind, unprompted by anything that had really occurred?

It took some work to convince David to return to the Senior Center. Periodically, the same theme would be repeated. The asshole had hit him in the head, beaten him up and no one was doing anything about it.

This reminded me of the bike that he thought I had stolen from him, the bike from 30 years ago. He was still quite convinced that I had stolen the bike. He was also convinced that I had thrown away his Navy P-coat from 30 years ago. He thought it should still have been hanging in the closet. Why wasn't it still hanging in the closet? Then there are all the CDs that he thinks I have stolen or that our daughters or grandson have stolen from him.

We are indeed into quite a bit of delusional thinking.

What David does try to accomplish is not very successful. I'm not sure that he realizes it, because he just keeps on doing it, no matter what the result is. He still tries to do the laundry, but he cannot differentiate between clean and dirty. He will fold the dirty clothes or leave everything in piles, then remark what a huge mess it is. The nicely folded dirty clothes sometimes make it back upstairs and into the bedroom before I realize that, in fact, they were never washed. I count it less as something that David can no longer do and more as something that I have to now pay more attention to. It's yet another task for me.

Once fastidious about the coffeemaker, David realizes that he has not been attentive to it, so he starts to take it apart. But he cannot wash the pieces of it and he cannot put it back together. He cannot make coffee. He cannot remember to tell me that he wants a cup of coffee, but he can take apart the coffee maker so that no one can get a cup of coffee until I figure out how to put it back together. Another task for me.

The status of dishes in the dishwasher is now always unknown, a mixture of clean and dirty, with glassware sitting precariously in the bottom rack. It's my first chore of the day now to clean out the dishwasher and start over. I also have to go through the garbage. Food and silverware get cleaned off the plates right into the garbage cans. Nothing can be taken for granted. I have to check and recheck everything.

He is eating huge amounts of ice cream, standing in front of the refrigerator with a big spoon in one hand and the half-gallon container in the other. Suddenly it makes me very sad. Suddenly I realize that he can no longer fix any food for himself and he does not let me know if he is hungry. So, he accesses what he likes and keeps on eating like a horse that doesn't know how to stop. His weight keeps climbing.

In the basement, David has taken out all of my father's old cameras and camera accessory pieces from a large old camera case. The pieces are strewn throughout the basement. He has also taken out all of the finely machined pieces to an expensive telescope that once belonged to his brother. These are also strewn throughout the basement. I don't recognize what pieces belong together. All I can do is retrieve them when I see them and put them in a drawer to deal with later.

There are so many things now in David's dresser drawers that the drawers will soon break. This includes his winter gloves, work gloves, two cameras, large pliers, screwdrivers and other tools, cards, magazines, pictures, CDs, hats, lots of wrapped and unwrapped coins, magazines and books. I know better than to touch his dresser, so I leave it all there and watch it grow.

✦ ✦ ✦ ✦ ✦ ✦

It's late January and our now nine-year-old grandson is lying down on the sofa with me sitting beside him. He is sick, so we are being quiet, watching TV. David comes up behind the sofa, saying, "So now you can tell me what you did with it. Are you going to tell me or not?" This is said in a seething, angry, grizzly-bear-like tone. He is grinding his teeth together as he speaks. He is now leaning over the sofa within inches of our grandson with the bottom end of some sort of meter that is missing the top part of it. He is using a very aggressive tone. "What did you do with it? Where is it?" I tell him to back off. Instead he starts jabbing the end of this object toward our grandson's arm. "I know you did it. Are you really going to just lie there and pretend you don't know anything about it?"

I am sometimes filling in words for David now, trying to fairly represent what he is saying, particularly when he's angry. That's when his speech comes haltingly. Words just seem to burst out of his mouth, but not necessarily in complete sentences. He repeats some words and leaves out others. He may have actually said, "I know you. You did. You. Are you really going to? You just lie there? You pretend. Don't know anything? Yeah, right! You don't know."

I tell him more forcefully to back off immediately. I tell him we do not have the meter. "Devon does not have the meter. We do not know anything about it. You will back off immediately!"

He does back off and stomps on down the hall, mumbling about how Devon has taken this thing, and I am protecting him (Devon). This disturbing episode occurred without any advance warning or sign. David had been quiet for hours and had been standing alone in the kitchen before this happened. He walked into the den and, within a few minutes, this interaction took place. It turned out that Devon, who was running a fever, had fallen asleep and luckily did not hear any of this... or so I thought. I found out later that Devon was purposely pretending to be asleep. Smart response, but sad that a nine-year-old has to deal with this. He is often the instigator, but on this day, he had had no interaction with David prior to this episode taking place. What must it feel like to have your sweet, loving grandfather turn on you like this?

I feel like I am so often lulled into complacency, when instead I need to be on the alert. When David is content, he is harmless, but I am seeing this growing disconnect between his anger and his ability to place the anger in context and deal with it in an adult manner. He is increasingly childish and unable to control his emotions.

✦ ✦ ✦ ✦ ✦ ✦

Last week, I saw the early-morning seizures come back. Again, everything is oh so temporary. David has been on seizure meds for many months now and it was good. There was so much improvement.

In the past, most of the morning seizure activity took the form of upper body jerks, the kind that caused him to inadvertently throw a cup of coffee across the room. Interesting that they used to happen when he was trying to hold something. They are not really seizures but uncontrolled body movements. Yet sometimes they are indeed seizures in that they affect him intellectually as well as physically. He zones out and I can't reach him.

This time, it happened when he was doing nothing more than patiently allowing me to dress him. His arm and shoulder flailed backwards. David was correspondingly unfocused the morning that this happened. It was difficult for him to understand simple instructions like "Give me your arm" (so I could put it in the sleeve of his shirt). I had missed one pill the day before. Usually this is not a problem if I miss a pill. Did my forgetfulness cause the seizure activity? I also noticed that over the past few nights, David has been having more of the minor nighttime jerking.

I want David to have a complete follow-up neuropsych exam again, just like the one that he had been given five years ago. I want to know where he is in this disease process. I also make a commitment to myself to aggressively pursue getting David seen by the VA system doctors. And if I can't make that happen right away, I will get him an appointment at McLean Hospital near Boston, which has been recommended to me a few times because it has a very good reputation for treating Alzheimer's patients and sorting out neurological problems.

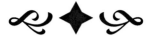

It's now March, not quite two months later, and today, David had a neuropsych exam by the same doctor who had evaluated him five years ago from the rehab hospital. I had set two goals. One was to pursue David's medical and potential long-term-care rights under the VA and the second was to pursue additional evaluations under our HMO medical insurance to see if there is anything else that we should be doing for him.

The first step with the VA was to get David enrolled. You have to be enrolled in the VA system to get any help at all, and there are gate guards to enrollment. While David is certainly eligible for medical services and reduced prescription costs, I knew that he would be at the very bottom of a long list of people eligible for long-term-care services from the VA, since his illness was not caused by or through his military service. Still, everything was worth the effort at this point. Since we had an HMO, I was not concerned with immediate care or prescription costs. It was the long-term care that was the real issue.

So I filled out the paperwork to enroll David, and we went to see our local VA rep to make sure that I had completed everything correctly. The rep reviewed it and said I had filled in everything correctly, and he explained that even soldiers coming back from Desert Storm were finding it difficult to get VA services. You really have to have a service-connected disability to get anywhere with potential long-term care. He also clearly indicated that there was no chance at all that an Alzheimer's diagnosis would be considered a service-connected disability.

That would never happen, despite the fact that David had served in Vietnam and been exposed to Agent Orange.

So, this just confirmed the information I already had. I sent in the application anyway and got no answer. Two months went by and I called, only to be told that David had been rejected by the VA and the paperwork was coming. Why? Well, he did not fit any of the categories of being destitute or having a service-connected disability of some acceptable percentage. I could have hung up the phone then, but I kept on talking, exasperated that someone like David, a career veteran with such an extreme illness, was being denied medical services. The lady said that I should call the director of the geriatric unit and talk to her about it.

I thought, *Why? You have already told me that he is rejected. What good will this do?* I felt like I was wasting my time, but I called and was put in touch with a social worker. She commiserated to a great degree about the limited services available through the VA. She went through each of the exclusion or inclusion categories for services and one that she mentioned was "catastrophic disability." I asked her what that meant and she said, "Well, that is a score on the Mini-Mental of less than 10, but of course you probably have no idea what this is."

"Oh no, I do know what that is," I shot back. "The Mini-Mental test? David has been given that test at least ten or twelve times."

She said, "Well, what was his last score?" I told her I thought it was a 14 or 15, maybe six to eight months ago. It had steadily dropped over the past several years, since we had started seeing a local neurologist.

The social worker said that scores can drop quite dramatically, and all patients suffering from Alzheimer's have good days and bad days. She advised me to always ask for the test when David sees any of his doctors or has any testing. She further advised me to tell the doctors not to help or cue David at all. "All he needs is a score of less than 10, and he will be eligible for VA long-term-care services." So this is what our support group members were trying to say to me so many times over. You have to push and push and push and never give up!

I mentioned to the social worker that we had this neuropsych exam coming up in a week. She said that the neuropsychologist probably will not administer the Mini-Mental unless I ask for it. It is not a sophisticated test, so they usually do not do it.

✦ ✦ ✦ ✦ ✦ ✦

Armed with this information, we showed up at the appointed time for David's second neuropsych exam. David greeted the psychologist warmly and seemed to remember her, although he probably didn't. I asked for the Mini-Mental test and explained why it was necessary. The doctor looked at both of us kindly and said she would be willing to give it to David, but I should know in advance that David's score would certainly not be less than 10. She smiled and said that less than 10 is quite extreme and David was not at that point. Still, she was willing to administer it.

The doctor took David into her office to start the tests. By midmorning, she came out to talk to me. She looked quite pale and serious. She had just given David the Mini-Mental test and told me quietly that he had scored a seven. She copied the results and signed them for me. I made a comment like "What people see when they look at David is deceiving. He is always smiling. They have no idea where he is with this disease." She agreed. David was not only less than 10, he was a seven. He was catastrophically disabled with points to spare!

With my new ammunition, I called back to the VA and was immediately invited to send all of David's records. I did that and got a notice back within a few weeks that he was to have an appointment at the VA hospital geriatrics unit in Bedford in August. It would be a six-month wait for that appointment, but at least and at last, we got the appointment. I felt triumphant!

The results of the neuropsych exam were not surprising. Where David still had strong verbal abilities five years ago, they now showed "significant decline." This time, he could not provide a writing sample at all. His visual integrative abilities were "severely impaired" as were processing speed, memory, working memory and executive functioning. "Mr. Brewer is close to the point where he may no longer be able to be cared for only by his wife." I was advised to start to look for additional help for David and some respite time for me. It was a negative-sounding milestone, but a milestone nonetheless. I knew exactly where we were in this journey.

✦ ✦ ✦ ✦ ✦ ✦

Not long after David's neuropsych exam, extra help came to us in a most unexpected way. Our nephew works at a local grocery store and happened to recognize one of the customers as David's good friend from the Coast Guard from many years ago. We knew Bernie and his family when we lived in Virginia. Our common bond was that both families planned to live on Cape Cod. After returning to the Cape, Bernie used to visit with David nearly every Sunday on his way to go shopping at the local military base. Some years later, we moved, and David and Bernie eventually lost touch.

A few phone calls later and we were back in touch. Bernie did not know that David was sick. He immediately offered to help me out on Thursdays, my day for taking care of Devon after school, so I could devote that time to Devon, and we could leave the house and separate ourselves from David. Bernie is now retired and this would give David and Bernie some time together. I was so grateful for this help.

Under the guise of entirely social calls, Bernie now spends time each week with David, and David seems comfortable, enjoying these visits. Sometimes Bernie brings a video or some music. He engages David, telling him about his family or bringing him up to date on what his old buddies from the Coast Guard are up to. Last month, he started taking David out for coffee, and this week they will be going up to the base to get a haircut. Bernie says he will take him each month up to the base to get a haircut. One less thing I have to think about. This is truly wonderful.

✦   ✦   ✦   ✦   ✦   ✦

It's April and I have gone through another strange period of being unable to write. I have not lacked for things to write about, but I find myself less able to capture what is happening. I can see, looking back, that each year I have written more and more and more. The significance of this experience is so much clearer to me now. The need to document it as it happens is something I obviously feel is very important because I have never read anything quite this detailed. If I had, it would have been helpful to me. I'm hopeful that this will be helpful to someone else.

Maybe right now, though, I am just too busy trying to live through it. Or, maybe I am just too much in a negative train of thought.

Last night, I thought seriously about divorcing David. I do not seem to be up to the job of taking care of him and, at the same time, remaining emotionally healthy. *Is it just a wild and crazy thought?* No, I really do have to think this through. Perhaps the court would appoint a caregiver for David, a guardian. Perhaps there is some way that I can be relieved of this burden in some positive way. *Would that be all right? What would people think of me if I did this?* It just sometimes feels like it is all too much.

✦ ✦ ✦ ✦ ✦ ✦

Once again, paranoia has turned into delusion. David has taken parts of things he recalls and put them together in a way that makes sense in his world of normal, and he truly, truly believes what he has constructed. The memory construct in turn becomes emotional, and emotion turns into aggressiveness, and aggressiveness explodes into anger and hatred. That is where we are. David hates Devon and he is dangerously angry and aggressive. The situation turns my stomach. *I no longer want to take care of David. I no longer want to live with David.*

About a week and a half ago, I noticed David picking up one of his ball caps and putting it down on the counter, shaking his head with a wry smile. He did this several times. It was enough to notice but not to worry about. He has lost all but two of his current supply of ball caps. All I thought at the time was, "Well, too bad. We'll need to get some more." This is not unusual. David loses things routinely.

At some point though, he turned to me and started in: "So you're telling me you don't know what happened to it?"

"What happened to what?"

"This...,"pointing at one of his ball caps. "Not this. The one I had with the round thing. The really nice round thing (drawing a circle with his hands). You know. Why are you acting so stupid? It's okay with you, isn't it? You let him steal my things and it's okay with you."

"What are you talking about?" I ask. I don't know why I ask because I can see that he is talking about a hat that he remembers, and I do know this particular hat that he remembers. I bought it for him in Bermuda and saved it to give to him at Christmas. He loved it. It had a colorful insignia on the front. Like many other hats, David lost it within a few weeks.

"Don't act like you're stupid. Are you really that stupid? I saw it. I SAW it."

By now, spit is starting to form on David's mouth as he yells and swings his arms around. His whole body is moving.

"Saw what? Who are you talking about?" I ask.

"Him. That boy. That little boy who comes here. You know. Don't act so stupid. Like you don't know. I SAW it. You don't believe me? Come here. I'll show you."

I go with David to the bedroom. He points to the top shelf in his closet. "There. That's where it was. I always put it there. Always. And he takes it. He steals from me and that's okay. You are really something, aren't you? You let it happen."

I tell David that there is no way that Devon would take his hat or want his hat or try to get something from the top shelf of his closet. No way. I told him that it sounds like he hates his own grandson. David says he wouldn't hate him if he did not steal from him every time he was in the house.

Now David starts following me around the house, repeating his angry accusations, continuing to flail his arms, getting more and more angry. I try ignoring him. I try distracting him. Finally, I hand him a Xanax, tell him to take it and tell him I'm leaving to go to the store, and that I hope that while I'm gone, he will simmer down and reconsider what he is saying about his grandson and how he is talking to me.

So, I leave for the store.

✦ ✦ ✦ ✦ ✦ ✦

It's the illness, illness, illness, not David. I repeat this mantra to myself, pounding on the steering wheel as I drive to the store, hoping that this little break from him will somehow allow me to detach from my feelings and restore my sanity. He wants me to hate him. No, he wants us all to hate him. It's crazy. This is not David. Not in any way, shape or form is this our David! David loves me. He loves our grandson. This is just not real.

Suddenly I'm enveloped in sadness as I flash back to the old David, the loving and kind David, the David who told me every single day how much he loved me. Always happy. Always smiling. I wouldn't have been driving to the store. It would have been David. He was always ready to run out to pick up the forgotten milk, a last-minute dinner item, or the Danish I suddenly couldn't live without. It didn't matter if it was 20 degrees out or 10 o'clock at night. He would have gone to the ends of the earth anytime just to find something really special for me.

He knew the store clerks by name from one end of town to the other. "Hi Jane!" he would grandly wave and yell across the front of Stop & Shop to reach a clerk at the very last register. Back would come a sea of waves and "Hi Dave's" as the various clerks would look up one by one, recognizing and welcoming him. I saw this happen over and over and never could quite fathom it. It was as though he had an invisible 10-gallon hat that exuded his southern charm. I couldn't have recognized a single one of these clerks, but David knew them all. This charming boy from Texas knew them all because people mattered to him, and he always had time for them, no matter who they were.

I'm sure other wives would be jealous to know how often David made dinner for both of us and then did the dishes afterwards. Then I might be sitting at my desk after dinner working through the bills, sometimes for hours. David was happy to leave me to the task of sorting out our finances. He knew his limitations! Still, he would come over to me with a gentle inquiry asking what I was working on and he would give me a kiss. Then suddenly a steaming cup of coffee would appear under my nose. He would follow that up later with more coffee and a warmed-up piece of apple pie or a brownie to help get me through the night.

I think about how our kids had such a great dad. When the girls were little, if it was my turn to get them to bed, I would resort to a fair amount of yelling in an effort to get them to quiet down. Not David. On his nights, he transformed into the prowling *go-to-sleep-monster* with hair-raising growls. "*BaaAAAHHHROOooo! BaaAAAHHHROOooo!*" He would run up the stairs and then lurk around their beds in the dark, waiting to pounce if they moved a muscle. They would be in hysterics hiding under the covers. In the mornings, out came *the-wakeup-pony*, a tiny little silver pony that he would lightly trot up and down their sleeping bodies, patiently waiting until they slowly opened their eyes.

Where is this sweet, kind, loving and patient man?

I think about how, not so long ago, he would have burst in the door after a long hot day out on the water working as an assistant harbormaster. His dog, Annie, would have jumped up on him with slobbering kisses, and he would have wrapped her in a big hug, telling her, "Annie, my love. What a wonderful dog you are. You are the best dog in the world."

Everything was in superlatives. As he tumbled his canvas satchel and thermos and lunch box onto the kitchen table, he would exclaim to me something like, "Oh I wish you could meet Mr. Ward. He is such a fantastic person and his boat! His boat is the most perfect, most beautiful boat in the bay. He keeps it shining from bow to stern. You should see it. It's really amazing. I really love this guy. His daughter is applying to the Coast Guard Academy, and, guess what? He asked me if I would write a letter of recommendation for her. Would I write a letter? You should meet her. She's so smart. I told him, of course, I would. I'd be honored. She's just what the Coast Guard needs. Can you believe it?" All this within the first minute of having arrived back home, eyes sparkling, grinning from ear to ear.

Where is this David? I know that he still exists within the person I left back at the house, but I can't find him and I miss him so much.

✦ ✦ ✦ ✦ ✦ ✦

My reverie abruptly ended when I returned home an hour later. David was still angry. He thought I had been gone for several hours and demanded to know exactly where I went, who I talked to, what I bought at the store. He criticized everything I brought home and then demanded his dinner.

Even the next day, his angry mood continued. I took him out to dinner hoping that he would start to feel better, but out of the blue after we ordered, David started in again.

"I thought they were leaving," he said in a sudden harsh and disgusted tone of voice.

"Who?" I asked.

"You know. The kids."

"Leaving. You mean moving?"

"You know what I mean," he growled at me.

"Well, yes," I reply. "They are planning to move, but not until next year." Kristin and Dennis would like to move further south, but they don't feel like they can do it now with David being ill.

"Will he be giving it back to me?" David asks.

"Giving what...?"

"Don't be stupid. You really are stupid, aren't you. Protecting him all the time. You think you are doing him favors, don't you. How do you think he'll turn out with you *ooh-ooh*ing all the time. You really are something." David's anger is apparent on his face. He is spouting out his words, and his face is getting red.

"You really and truly hate him, don't you?" I ask.

"You would too if he stole your stuff," David replies.

"He didn't steal your stuff. He doesn't deserve your hate."

"Prove it. Go on. Prove it. You can't. You can't deny the truth. I know he stole it from me and (fist on the table, eyes getting watery, red-faced) he had no right. He had no right to steal from me."

This, of course, destroyed our dinner out. I could not even look at David and we left quickly after. Going out to dinner had been one thing that we could still do together and have a bit of a happy time. This exchange in public made it obvious that we would probably not be going out to dinner anymore.

At some point, I looked at David and saw someone who is unreachable. I just can't find that wonderful person he used to be anymore. I'm not sure that Devon should ever come back to our house. Devon will sense this hostility immediately. I hate being put in this position. I thought we had gotten past this stage of his illness. If I am forced to choose, I will choose Devon. So then what would happen? Do I just clean out a bank account, pack up my stuff and go rent some place to live without looking back? Does that dump David into the laps of our two daughters? They very clearly have stated their position with regard to his aggressiveness and abusiveness. They will not stand for it. Can we all turn our backs on him and walk away? It feels like a heinous crime just to be thinking along these lines.

✦ ✦ ✦ ✦ ✦ ✦

Spring is bursting out all over. The grass looks good, thank God. It's warm and lovely.

David's doctor responded to his aggressiveness by prescribing him a double dose of Xanax to be given to him whenever necessary. He also now takes 60 milligrams of Paxil daily. I noticed that when I happened to give him a dose of Paxil around the same time as a dose of Xanax, he was actually subdued and withdrawn for a while. This will now be the routine pre-med whenever Devon is due to visit us. I don't like playing doctor in this way, and I am beginning to wonder when David will max out his meds and there will be no medical solution left. But for now, we are back to an even keel.

Bernie has been coming faithfully on Thursdays, and while David sometimes asks why he comes, he seems to continue to enjoy his time with Bernie. He is certainly glad to have another guy to talk to, instead of me.

We went out for pizza with Kristin and Devon and Dennis. David was mostly well behaved and cooperative, but not very talkative. The ball game was on three wall TVs. At one point, David picked up on the sports atmosphere, stood up and grabbed his crotch. Kris could have slunk under the table when she saw her dad do this.

He seems wide awake this morning at 6:00 a.m., which is unusual but part of the pattern of unpredictable behavior. The radio was on to wake me up. I have to go to work. David announced that he couldn't understand what they were saying on the radio. The words were vague. Everyone was vague. He told me I was real, but everyone else was vague. I can hear him now in the bathroom. He probably thinks this is a school day, but it's not. He calls his Day Center "going to school." How will David get on in this house all morning all by himself? I feel that I have no choice but to leave for work; it makes me very worried.

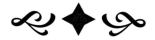

Midsummer. David is in a bad mood. What else is new? He slept all night and all the next day from 11:00 p.m. Friday to 6:00 p.m. Saturday. After being up for about three hours, he said something about a camera being missing. This was a guess based on the few clues that David gave me as to why he was upset. I figured out that he was commenting about a very old camera that had belonged to my father.

"You guys are getting fucked. You can't see it (lots of sneering). He just smiles. He's got that way and you guys are suckers. He looks at me like this (mimics a sly grin). You don't see it, so just forget it. You guys will never get it."

Translated, this jumble of words alludes to our grandson who David believes has stolen the very old camera belonging to my father. Devon, of course, has never touched the camera. He has no interest in old things.

A week later. Again, David is in a bad mood, or maybe he is still in a bad mood. I'm not sure if he ever gets out of his bad moods anymore.

Today, David went to the Day Center. In the evening, he tells me that there is someone at his center who needs help, so he is going to help her. Maybe he will marry her. It's a woman. No, he corrects himself. Maybe it was her mother. But in any case, she has nothing. She does not have the military. She has nothing. No one to help. So he thinks he will marry her to give her the help from the military. But oh, he is already married, so he does not think that he can do that. He says he will talk to the person who knows all about this.

✦ ✦ ✦ ✦ ✦ ✦

We have a new problem. David says that Bernie is trying to convert him. Bernie took David on a drive and stopped at his church, the Catholic church in Brewster, Our Lady of the Cape. Both Bernie and his wife are active in the church. The church has a beautiful large addition, and Bernie wanted to show it to David. He thought it might make a nice outing for David to drive down to Brewster to see the new church wing. David is convinced, though, that this is part of a plan to convert him and that the sole reason that Bernie comes over to our house is that he is trying to convert David to Catholicism. Otherwise, what reason did he have to come over?

David repeated this same theme many times to Kristin and Dennis while we were sitting on the porch. They tried to convince David that Bernie is his friend and cares about him. He does not care about converting him. David laughed scornfully at this. He remains convinced otherwise. Poor Bernie, who is so kind to David! He cannot escape the paranoia any more than we can.

✦ ✦ ✦ ✦ ✦ ✦

Over the past weekend, David sunk into a really black mood. It was prompted by my allowing Dennis to borrow David's truck. Eventually I was able to permanently hide the truck keys from

David. While he would grumble from time to time about not being able to drive, he seemed to accept it for the most part. His truck sits on the other side of the house unused except for when I drive it to the dump on Sundays. Dennis also has a truck, but it was overheating. So he parked it in our driveway and, *with my permission,* he borrowed David's truck. I did tell David that I had given Dennis permission to borrow his truck.

The next day, David looked out the window and saw Dennis's truck in our driveway. His conclusion was that Dennis had an evil plan to swap trucks so that he (Dennis) would not get any scratches on his own truck. Dennis's evil plan was to abuse and ruin David's truck and the rest of us were all in cahoots with him. To further aggravate the situation, Dennis has not called a tow truck yet. So this same theme has been repeated many, many times each day over the past six or so days that David's truck has been gone. Each time, David's face takes on a scowling look of bitter hatred. I finally called Dennis and told him that this is causing a problem and would he please call a tow truck to move his truck out of the driveway, get it repaired, and get David's truck back home.

When the weekend came, David once again rejected me as his caregiver, throwing some of my things out of our bedroom. He told me that I was selfish, and since I had taken over the guest bedroom with my sewing machine and my cello, he was now taking over our bedroom. He placed a chair behind the door but it didn't prevent me from getting the door open. I was able to get in and found him asleep in the middle of the day. He slept nearly 48 hours straight. As I thought about it, there was nothing else he could have done; he was in such a bleak and angry mood. He was too angry and too depressed to be awake.

✦ ✦ ✦ ✦ ✦ ✦

This is getting very tough to take as we are now in mid-summer, and David continues to be in a very bad mood. While standing in the garage, he points to the barn plaque that Kristin painted for us as a gift and says in a very gruff tone, "That was a big lie. Wasn't it? Wasn't it? A big lie." His face turns to a tight grimace and remains that way for the rest of the night. Kristin painted this for our new barn, the one at the old house, now sold. Sold because it was not compatible with David's illness. Sold and gone. Sad. I'm sad. David is angry.

Later he comes through the doorway of the kitchen with his head bent low. He says, "So what was that all about trying to get these things out of my head. These bugs. See? Do you see them? What? You don't see them? You're pretending that you don't know?"

"Well, let me show you," he continues. "Come with me. Come and I will show you."

He grabs my arm and leads me to his bathroom where he picks up the face cleanser that I had purchased for him. "Here it is. It's right here," he says.

I explain that the cleanser is to help clear up his nose. It has nothing to do with his head. But he laughs derisively at this. I point to his nose and tell him that he has had a lot of acne popping out on his nose because of his medications. "This medicine works very well to keep it under control," I explain.

David scowls and says, "No. Oh no. That's not it!" He tells me that I gave it to him. That is, I gave him the skin problems. He never had a problem with it before. Never. So his conclusion is that I gave the acne to him.

Then he looks in the mirror. "Where is the acne? Where? Do you see it?" he asks. "It's not there, is it?"

I tell him that I have had him wash his face with this cleanser, and it has improved his skin, so he does not have as bad a problem with it as he did before. The cleanser has helped him. Again he laughs derisively and he keeps on laughing for what seems to me to be a long time.

Sometimes I can't tell if I am goading him in some way, maybe leading him on, or am I actually being reasonable with him, trying to minimize his anxiety? I'm sure he feels my impatience.

✦   ✦   ✦   ✦   ✦   ✦

The weather has been so hot and humid. I took David and Devon to the lake for a swim. Devon promised to be good. That is, not instigate things with David. Each time we attempt to do anything with David now, I have to give Devon a prep talk.

Aah, but he just couldn't resist this time. So Devon happily splashed David repeatedly once we were in the water. I watched with trepidation as Devon had the air mattress in one arm and was splashing David with the other. David's response was to tear away the air mattress from Devon's grasp and then throw it up on the beach.

The angry moment passed, but then it was like déjà vu. Later, when Devon and I both had our air mattresses in the water, not splashing David at all, David angrily made his way to us in the water and tore both of the air mattresses away from us. He stormed up to the beach where he threw the air mattresses down, gritting his teeth and angrily complaining about Devon's behavior. Devon was agape, wondering what had just happened.

I told David to control himself or I would call the police. Eventually, he left the beach on his own and waited for us in the parking lot.

Later, Devon and I were rinsing off in the outside shower. David was just outside the shower door yelling about Devon using his soap. He suddenly slammed the shower door hard against me in an attempt to grab Devon. When I expressed surprise that he would hurt me to get to Devon, he said it was my own fault and "too bad." I don't know what set him off, but I do know now that once David feels anger, it can come out in unexpected ways and at unexpected times. How can I stay one step ahead of him?

✦　✦　✦　✦　✦　✦

For several months now, there has been some improvement in David's level of seizure activity. David's neurologist increased his dose of Depakote at bedtime and that seems to have done the trick. While his anger and depression have been particularly difficult to live with, otherwise, we have been doing well. He has been attending the Day Center two days a week. We have been walking and swimming, running errands. I've been able to focus on my job, so, all in all, things have been going well.

One day in August, when I went into the bedroom late in the morning to get David up, I found him already sitting on the side of the bed waiting for me. I helped him to get dressed, and then we went into the bathroom to get him washed and shaved. David pointed to his wedding ring, remarking about how tight it was getting. I agreed with him. While I was holding his hand in the sink and thinking that we will have to do something soon about his rings, a major seizure suddenly gripped David.

He grunted as it crumpled him and sent him crashing to the floor. He would have struck the ceramic tile floor very hard but somehow I caught him in midair under one arm and slammed my body against him so as to hold him up. Then I slid my head and shoulders under his left arm, grabbed that arm with my left arm and slid my right arm around his back, reaching out and grabbing for his right arm, tucking it against his chest. Somehow in this grab and hold, I was able to slide him toward the side of the bed and sit him down.

My first thought was *Damn, and we were doing so well.* David's body continued with minor jerking afterwards. Everything seems precarious after these episodes. I made him sit there and not get up for a while. When I thought he could be safe enough, I ran to the kitchen, put some coffee in a mug with a lid, brought it to him and gave him some sips. Maybe coffee would wake him up a bit more, get him out of this sleep-to-wake zone that is so hard for him.

This time, there did not seem to be any accompanying loss of focus, but it was physically draining for both of us. If this was not a seizure, it was certainly a lightning strike and very, very dangerous. The chances of him splitting his head open while alone when one of these occurs would be huge. Why does something always tip the equilibrium the other way, just when I get to thinking that things are under control?

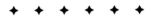

David is binge eating despite the fact that I have been giving him extra food to keep him satisfied. His dinner, half of my dinner, leftovers, ice cream, more ice cream, and then more ice cream. He can't stop. I have to disengage him and clear away all traces of food, or it will go in his mouth.

When he ate an entire cherry torte that I had worked on half the day, it was too much for me. I reacted emotionally. *How could he do this to me?* I rarely cooked. My cherry torte was a masterpiece! I was so proud of myself. When I returned to the kitchen, there it was...a few crumbs and the empty pan. I am so disgusted and so disappointed and so sad and so empty. His response was that I don't feed him and the Day Center doesn't feed him, so I deserved it!

I feel like I don't exist anymore. *I don't exist. I am invisible and nonexistent.*

He tells me that I get the best of everything and he gets nothing. He thinks that Dennis, Kristin and Devon are methodically stealing from him. He tells me that I am pathetic and too stupid to see what they are doing.

I can feel a growing resentment that this illness is taking too long to evolve to the next stage—the one where David becomes more accepting and more complacent, the one where maybe he will just forget who I am and, with that forgetfulness, he will no longer own the jealousy factor or the paranoia that has characterized him for so much of this year. It is wearing me out in so many ways. Or, maybe he will truly get violent, and then someone else will have to step in to control him.

I just want to be done with this. I know it is a long road ahead, but I just want to be done with it, and I have no idea how I will continue to cope.

✦ ✦ ✦ ✦ ✦ ✦

It's been another particularly difficult and troubling morning with David. I woke him up at the usual time. He'd had his usual pills the day before. Nothing was out of the ordinary except that after he went to the bathroom, he came back to the side of the bed and stood there. I pointed to his clothes laid out on the other side of the bed and indicated that he should come and sit down so he could get dressed.

David just stood there, ignoring me. I again pointed to his clothes and asked him to please come and sit down so I could help him get dressed. "Yup" was all he said, but he did not move at all. He was staring straight ahead.

I waited a minute more and tried again. No response. It seemed at first that David was being difficult and uncooperative, standing his ground. Then I realized that he was in a seizure, in some kind of zone where he simply could not respond to me. I walked up to him and looked closely into his face. His eyes were unfocused. Once again, I tried to coax him to the side of the bed to sit down. He started to hum in a pattern. Three hums, then silence for two seconds, then three hums again. He did this over and over for about 10 minutes.

Scared of what might happen next, I grabbed David's arm forcibly and guided him to the side of the bed where he could sit down. As he walked, he started to have very mild tremors. As I held on to him, I could feel him start to lurch forward. I was very afraid that he would fall. I commented to him, "You are not focused today, are you?"

There was no answer. I repeated it and he answered, "No."

I said, "You are having a difficult time today, right?"

He responded, "Yes."

We finally made it to the bed and I got him to understand that he needed to lie back on the pillows for a while until this fog went away. It took another 15 minutes, so altogether this period of awake-unconsciousness lasted about 30 minutes. He continued with very minor tremors during this time. Even later into the day, he needed extra instructions and more support than usual.

I had to guide him to the back porch for lunch, guide him into his chair, help him to pick up his sandwich, remind him to keep eating.

What is happening? We are once again into a period of instability. He is more confused in the bathroom. If I leave the toothpaste out, he will put it on his face. If he successfully puts shaving cream on his face, he then tries to shave his face with his electric toothbrush. I don't know why I am surprised when these things happen, but I am. No sooner do I figure out how to deal with something or get medications changed and stabilized than we are into some new challenge that has to be met. It's clear that David needs constant supervision when he is about to get up in the morning, and certainly when he is awake and moving about the house.

I am not able to keep up with this supervision. I listen for his footsteps. I check on where he is and what he is doing a hundred times a day. And still, it doesn't seem to be enough. I am also feeling guilty because I realize that I fell asleep early last night and forgot to give him his last Depakote for the day. *Will he have difficulty waking up today? Will he have seizures because of my forgetfulness?* I have now set an extra clock to ring an alarm at night, so I can be sure to give David his pills.

✦ ✦ ✦ ✦ ✦ ✦

We had our first appointment at the VA hospital in Bedford this week. It took about two hours to get there. Since it was early in the morning, I had to get David ready and out of the house at 5:00 a.m., which was no small feat. I explained to David where we were going, telling him that I thought it was important that we make sure that he is getting the best care. With his military service, he deserves whatever the VA has to offer. He seemed to understand, or perhaps he was disinterested, or perhaps it was just all beyond his capability to understand. Hard to tell.

The hospital, with its many imposing red brick buildings, sat on beautiful grounds. I found the right set of offices, but noticed that there was a medical meeting of some sort going on in a conference room that we could see through glass windows. I sat David down in the waiting room. After about 20 minutes, someone called my name and I looked up to see the conference room people all lined up in the hallway, looking at us. There was a doctor, two interns, two social workers and a nurse. Someone said, "We're ready for David now."

I looked at them, not quite believing this. I stammered, "Are you all here for David?"

"Yes," someone replied. They all were. There were nods of acknowledgment, and introductions were made around the group. David smiled at each and every one and shook their hands. One of the assistants was going to take David to another room, and I was to join everyone else in the conference room.

I couldn't help it, I guess. Tears started running down my face. All these people were taking this kind of time to help us? It was unreal.

For a few hours, I was questioned as to David's status, his skills and lack of skills, his personality, the anger and aggressiveness, the seizure activity, his medications. It didn't take much for me to spew forth all that had been happening.

Then I was invited to visit one of the two Alzheimer's wings with one of the social workers. I told her how amazed I was at the reception. She said that they were like a family there, and that David was now considered part of that family. They would be doing everything possible to help him. When it came time for him to enter long-term care, he would be accepted. My immediate response was "You're kidding. That's amazing. What about the cost?"

She told me that there is a financial review, and I would likely pay something, but it wouldn't be a lot. She told me that the VA does not make spouses destitute. Further, I would not have to contribute my retirement savings toward David's care. This seemed too good to be true.

Then we visited the Alzheimer's wing. I knew it would be a lockdown unit, but behind those locked doors, it seemed confined and stuffy, almost claustrophobic. Some beds were in small alcove rooms and some were in a larger shared room. There were several patients in wheelchairs in a circle where they were being encouraged to participate in some chair exercises. Almost no one did, though. I told the social worker that I couldn't imagine David being there. I wanted to leave. She said that she understood, and it was a very normal first reaction.

During this time, the doctor met with David. We were to all meet up again after lunch to continue the interviews. But when we did meet again, it was just for a short period of time. The doctor told me that David was not a candidate for long-term care at this time and really did not seem to want to give me any more help or direction than that. He said that obviously, David is too socially aware and too socially intact to confine to their long-term-care program. It would be akin to cruel and unusual punishment. He would make some recommendations regarding David's medications and send those to his neurologist.

I realized so many things right at that point in time. David had been so engaging when he said "Hello" to everyone in the hallway, just like he always is. He had happily and willingly followed one of the medical assistants to a private little room where I could hear him immediately take up a rousing conversation regarding the beautiful weather. He was probably quite jovial with the doctor when the doctor interviewed him. So, I totally agreed that David was not yet a candidate for their long-term care. That wasn't a surprise. I didn't bring David to the VA to be admitted. I wanted their care and counsel and advice. I wanted to find out about long-term care for the future, not for now.

What was a big surprise was the certain knowledge that David's intact social skills and youthful good looks were going to work against him, and probably already had. How many people did we know who really couldn't acknowledge that the laughing, smiling, joking David was actually sick? How many people had no idea that behind closed doors, David was a different person and saved the worst for his family?

Of course, the doctors had reviewed his medical information and based on that and based on his score of seven on the Mini-Mental test, automatically qualifying him as catastrophically disabled, he would certainly be ready for their long-term-care unit. But then they saw him face to face and interacted with him and came to a different conclusion.

There was the rub. David was not socially catastrophically disabled. His social skills, at least with people outside our family, were still excellent. For the most part, illness did not show on David's face.

It was clear to me that it would be a long time before David would be considered a proper candidate for long-term care.

For me, it meant that I was caring for a person who, for all intents and purposes, should be in a skilled nursing facility but smiled too much to be admitted. We were told to come back in six months. I was worried about the level of continuing care that David would need during the interim. How can I ever do enough to provide what he needs?

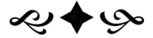

It was a good summer, yet it was also an unstable and unpredictable time. Now we're into the fall, and we are very clearly in a different place. This disease has advanced itself, reached a plateau and then grasped on full force once again to effect more changes.

Overall, David just seems more zoned out for longer periods of the day. He is more childlike and dependent. Faucets are left on. The shower was left on for hours before I found it along with tile damage and a big lake in the basement. David denied that he did it. Why would he do that? Of course it wasn't him!

He is frustrated by his inability to put a sentence together at times. He will remark about something and be quite excited by whatever he is thinking, but about 50 percent of the time now, he cannot get the idea across to me, and he just gives up with a huff.

Eating continues to be a problem, with David gorging on food in the kitchen, saying that he is starved and that I never feed him. Making him extra meals to try to meet his hunger level is a logical response to an illogical problem. He is not really hungry. He just cannot remember when he last ate, and food being a most basic human necessity is something that he still understands and thinks he can control.

David moves very slowly and is very sensitive—everything is an inconvenience or an interference. He can barely fit himself into the front seat of the car. It's not his size. It's his lack of coordination. It's becoming a major ordeal for him to avoid hitting his head on the top of the car or his arm on the door. If he does bump himself, he says *Ow* in a childish voice and rubs whatever hurts like he will never recover. Sometimes, when I lead him around, I realize that I am pulling on him and he says it hurts. I hate it when I realize that I am leading him around like a dog, but I can't seem to get him to move.

Noises hurt him too. He cringes in pain when I slam a car door, and it's real pain. I can see that. It really hurts him, so I try to be careful. I try not to make any loud noises.

Although I fully realize that I am totally responsible for his safety, I have given up trying to encase him in a seatbelt. While driving, I imagine the defense I will give a police officer if we are stopped. "Yes, I understand that it is state law to wear a seat belt, but my husband has Alzheimer's Disease and he will not cooperate with me. He is just having too much difficulty in physically adjusting himself into a car, let alone getting a seat belt positioned over him. And, and, and…it just takes too much time!" Part of me hopes that I will be found irresponsible, and some officer will lead us into court before a judge, and I will stand up to take my punishment, but they will take David away to be better cared for somewhere else, and that will be okay with me.

✦ ✦ ✦ ✦ ✦ ✦

Now we have a new challenge. Swallowing pills is apparently going to quickly become a thing of the past. David puts pills in his mouth and rolls them around. He does not understand how to swallow pills anymore, although he is able to swallow food. Is he being willful? He can take a drink of water without swallowing the pills in his mouth. How does he do that? Sometimes I find a pill in there half an hour later if I don't remember to check his mouth right away. I tell him to swallow, and I make gulping sounds like an idiot over and over, but David does not seem to be able to understand me at all.

I swath my finger all over the inside of his mouth looking for the pills, risking his biting my finger off. Sometimes I find a pill and sometimes I don't. I am not getting whether or not this is part of a new physical limitation. Again, the alarm bells sound in my heart. I have read about swallowing difficulties. That spells real trouble if that is what is going on.

✦ ✦ ✦ ✦ ✦ ✦

I am now quite convinced that David will have a serious injury in the bathroom. It is just a question of when it will happen. How do I prepare for it, other than to be so unfathomably stressed out with listening for any little thing that can go wrong in an instant?

In the mornings, he is having uncontrolled bowel movements— maybe that's the beginning of incontinence. I don't know how incontinence starts. Shouldn't I know that? All the books I have read do not go into the particulars. It's not exactly diarrhea. More like he has held it in and held it until…it explodes out of him.

Then maybe once every one to two weeks in the very early morning around 4 or 5 a.m., David gets himself into the

252

bathroom and realizes what a mess he has made, but at the same time that this occurs, he is in seizure mode. He cannot understand what I say to him. He cannot do what I tell him to do. He, in fact, refuses to be helped and tries to push me away. Then the seizure lurching starts.

So here we have David with his dirty hands and towel, poop in the sink, poop in his jammies and underwear, on his butt, down his legs, eyes bulging, body twitching and body lurching. I command him over and over and over to please sit on the toilet, but he will not do it. Instead, he stands there trying to touch things, picking up a toothbrush, not knowing at all what he is doing, twitching and lurching. I run out, unwilling to watch him crash to the floor. Then I come back, then I run out again. *What is wrong with me that I can't handle this? What to do? What to do?*

Eventually, I get lots of towels and start to lay them all around us, over the sink, on the floor, on the carpet, on the bed. I use several to clean him up as I pull him out of his dirty clothes. While holding him upright to prevent him from lurching to the floor, I push and pull him back to the bed. Then, when David is clean and comfortable, I have to wash the two rugs, eight towels, the sink, the floor and the toilet, while David goes back to sleep. After washing everything down, I disinfect it with Clorox.

Part of me thinks that I cannot handle this myself simply because it is such a difficult mess for me, not because it is a physical danger to David. I don't think I have been truly tested yet. *Or maybe this is the beginning of being truly tested. Maybe this is the beginning of when do I reach my limit? When does David reach a reasonable limit with my ability to protect him? When does all of this outweigh the importance of our marriage and our time together? Who can help me with this? I am so alone...*

✦ ✦ ✦ ✦ ✦ ✦

There is a bewilderment and anger at play in David's paranoia that becomes so much more complicated by his painfully limited communication ability at times. Sometimes I think no one else could possibly understand him. The angrier he gets, the less intelligible his communications become. Yet oddly, I can understand him. Every word. Every nuance.

I have been so shocked by his growing verbal limitations that, at times, I have rushed off to write down exactly what I heard. This was what David had to say one night when I was getting him ready to go to bed:

"These guys. They're coming to get me. Ha ha ha. They get... They're all like ha ha ha. Oohweeeeee! Got him! That's why he comes here. Selling me. Trying to sell me. You can't do that. You can't speak for yourself? Good God, Sonja. I thought you were more than that. You used to be. I don't need you. Ha ha ha. I'll talk. I will not talk to anyone. How's that? That's mine. You can't take it (making sucking sounds with his nighttime pills in his mouth). I'm not getting anyone to me. Yeah, go ahead. They'll think you're crazy. Just consider that I'm not doing anything like that. I'm zero. Nothing. Blah blah blah, that's all I'm hearing (now walking away from me, taking the pillows out of the room with him, presumably to go sleep elsewhere). Just tell him can't do it. Don't want to do it."

I had to go get David and lead him back to the bedroom, lay him down in the bed and put the covers over him. Responding to this would be stupid on my part. My job is to minimize his agitation, comfort him, help him to go to sleep.

I knew exactly what was causing this agitation and what he was trying to say. His paranoia is climbing to new heights. He is so convinced that his friend Bernie is trying to convert him to Catholicism that his entire friendship with Bernie is on the line. David says that the church needs money and so that is why Bernie is still so determined to come over every week to work so hard at converting him. I keep telling David over and over that Bernie is his good friend. He comes to spend time with him because he is his friend.

I remind David that Bernie comes over to take him to Dunkin' Donuts for coffee and Bernie takes him to the base to get a haircut. Bernie brings him music CDs and videos. Did that sound like someone who wanted to harm him? David shakes his head, "No," but continues to scowl. His face is contorted and angry. When he becomes so singularly focused on being agitated and angry, he can't easily let go and relax. He certainly can't sleep. He finally rolls over in the bed, but continues to scowl, saying things under his breath that seem to start and end with "You people…" He whips the covers over his head.

✦ ✦ ✦ ✦ ✦ ✦

It's now October and David had a few medical appointments last week. One was with his urologist who is following David for an enlarged prostate. His PSA level is up a bit. I had to take him for blood work the week before. David is very cooperative with these ventures, although he has no idea why we are doing them. As long as I stop for coffee, he is generally happy. At the lab, I stay by David's side, answer the questions that are repeatedly asked of him. I want to say, *Don't you remember that he does not remember his birth date? You should remember that. Don't be distracted by his pleasant manner and his quick smile. This is an ill person. Why can't you remember that?*

I get mixed results asking David what he feels. Does he have trouble urinating? It seems to me that he waits a long time to go. Sometimes he says yes; sometimes he says no. Most of the time I don't think he understands the concern. The doctor said that his enlargement is firmer now; and he wants to do a second biopsy in December. The first one was done about two years ago and it came out fine. David wondered why we were at this doctor's office and I tried to explain. He looked at me blankly. I can't imagine what it must be like to have a major illness along with Alzheimer's Disease. How do you cope? It's like having a small child with a major illness. You just never know what to take seriously.

The second appointment was with David's neurologist. This time, I told the doctor that David's pill-swallowing difficulties were now extreme. He would no longer be able to take pills. The doctor very patiently looked up each medication and was able to replace all of them with dissolvable or liquid forms. I've been waiting about a week now for the mail-in orders to be delivered. Meanwhile, it's excruciating to get David to swallow a pill. I have to hang on to him, watch him, cajole him, demonstrate it to him, give him water. Sometimes he just gets mad at me, and then it's even more difficult.

Apparently, swallowing is a learned reflex. Odd that we have to learn something that is necessary to keep us alive! The difficulty is forgetting or apraxia. David is forgetting how to swallow. Well, if that is the case, then it would seem that eating food or drinking liquids will also become problems. Why just the pills? I have been watching David more closely. In fact, he has been leaving drinks behind at the table. Coffee, water, soda, juice. All of it. We always used to keep 20-ounce cups around for David because he would drink like a crazy person all day long. Not drinking is very unusual for him.

Kris told me that at the nursing home where she worked, they would put some kind of thickener into the drinks for people in the Alzheimer's unit because they had trouble swallowing. *What? Why haven't I ever heard about this before, with all I have read about this illness? Crazy!* One day, I experimented. When David did not drink his water, I put a straw in it and handed it to him. He sucked it right down. Hmmm... Sucking trumps lips on a glass! But for how long?

David can still use a fork and spoon quite well, but both are used for scooping a lot. Sometimes he just uses the spoon and a finger to scoop up rice and pieces of meat. I realize that he has been using his hands a lot, and he's very messy, taking apart sandwiches before eating them. He never used to do that before. *What is the point? Is he trying to make bite-sized pieces?* The other night, he tore his pizza slices into small pieces. I wondered if the pizza crust was too hard for him to chew and swallow. I will have to keep watching.

I also told the neurologist that I am not satisfied with David's seizure control. How and when I got to this point, where I have now fully taken over all aspects of David's medical care, I am not sure. I don't know. It just happened. I now have no qualms about being ultra direct with his doctors.

I explained the morning episodes, the bowel incontinence combined with seizures (a combination that has occurred quite a few times so far) plus other episodes of early-morning seizures that occur in the bedroom or bathroom. I made it very clear that this time of day is the only time when I feel that I cannot control the situation. I encircle David with my arms to prevent him from lurching to the floor. Sometimes he is focused during these attacks, but most of the time he is unfocused and unable to comprehend anything I say to him; he is unable to follow directions. This puts us both at risk. The other change is that sometimes David appears to be fine when he gets up, then he zones out half an hour later, and then the jerking and lurching starts. I have to be ever so vigilant. It now means that I have to get him up earlier on the days when he goes to the Day Center in Orleans, because I have to manage his morning routine with such deliberate slowness.

So, we have another increase in the dosage of Depakote. Of course, since I find the pills spat out or not taken, he is not up to the level he is supposed to be at until we get the dissolvable form of Depakote.

✦ ✦ ✦ ✦ ✦ ✦

Next week, we hit the next milestone. I will have a PCA in to take care of David so I can go to orchestra rehearsal on Wednesday night. Kris has been helping me out the last two Wednesdays.

I just can't leave David alone anymore. He gets too anxious and it is too dangerous. So, it will cost me my day's pay to get a PCA, but that is the general direction we are heading in, and there's really nothing I can do about it. I can't focus on the money end of things. That is about the farthest thing from my mind right now.

✦ ✦ ✦ ✦ ✦ ✦

Another delusion yesterday. David pointed to our neighbor's house and remarked about all the work they were doing. I said, "What work?"

He said, "See? See the sand? Don't you see all the sand?"

"No," I replied. "There is no sand and nothing is going on over there. You are looking at their roof." The shingles on this house are orange and brown.

"No," David says. "You don't know what you're talking about. All that sand. They've been working on that house a long time. You really don't know what's going on around here, do you?"

I then exploded. "David, I'm sorry but there is nothing going on at that house, nothing being built, no sand, no sand at all, no sand anywhere. You are wrong. You are seeing things that don't exist, and I have to tell you that there is NO SAND over there. BELIEVE ME!"

David then pointed to the ground and told me that of course there is sand everywhere we look—on the ground, in their yard, in our back yard, everywhere. He didn't mean just over at that house. Of course he didn't mean just over at that house. Whatever gave me that idea? I gave up at this point. We have no sand in our back yard. It's dirt and grass. Brown dirt and green grass. So why is he seeing sand? Then he realizes that he is not seeing sand at all, or maybe by now, he is embarrassed about seeing sand when there is no sand?

Why do I take it upon myself to argue with him? Why do I do that?

A few days later, while enjoying the last of the fall's warm days on our porch, David pointed to the tops of the pine trees. "Look at all that sawdust."

"What are you talking about?" I ask him, trying to look in the direction where he is looking, up at the expanse of tall pines that encircle our back yard. There is nothing unusual there. The sunlight of the late afternoon highlights the tops of the trees. There is only sunlight where he sees sawdust on the treetops. I say nothing.

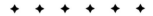

I had been advised somewhere along the way to contact our local Elder Services, that they offer services for residents with Alzheimer's Disease. The first call was unsuccessful. I was told that their services are for people who are at least 60 years old. I mentioned what I had been told about services for Alzheimer's patients to no avail. They could not help.

Again, the topic of local resources came up at our support group, and again I was told that Elder Services provides help to Alzheimer's patients. So, I made the call again and yet a different person told me the same thing. No help. I then said that I had been told quite clearly that residents under the age of 60 with an Alzheimer's diagnosis were eligible for services, and I asked to speak to a supervisor or director. The person got off the phone and came back and suddenly said she would take down some of my information, and a caseworker would contact me. I am learning to push back.

The caseworker conducted an at-home interview with me for over an hour. David passed through the room, smiled and shook her hand and asked how she was doing. He was impressive as he always is. She seemed to understand that this illness and David's pleasant personality could actually cohabitate in the same human body. Someone who understood this illness, even a fractional part of it, was something relatively new for me. I found it therapeutic to just sit and talk to her, to help her fill in what David could do and could not do. To determine what stage David is at in the disease process. It seemed very clear that he was at mid-stage, maybe even late mid-stage.

In the end, there were no services available to us. Our combined incomes put us above the threshold for help. At this point, our combined incomes had dropped over $50,000 due to this disease, which was a significant drop for us, but we were not yet at poverty level. I inquired how people living on Cape Cod under their income threshold could possibly pay a mortgage and buy groceries. She assured me that she did not know, but of course, most of the people that Elder Services helped were actually elderly and did not have mortgages. Well that would explain a lot. It's the double whammy, of course! An old person's disease at a young age.

She said she would see me again in a few months. I now had an open case file, even though I had no eligibility for paid services. She did, however, provide an extraordinary resource for me and, in fact, assured me that it was okay to take advantage of such a resource. It was so simple and yet something that I would not have done for myself until I was at wits' end. She arranged for a personal shopping service to purchase my groceries for me. I had to pay for the service, but it was so worth it. I sat down at my computer and drew up a master plan for standard meals and a list of the things that I always buy: a core of products that would see us through up to two weeks if we were on a desert island. It became my standard list, and we started to eat plain and simple food, nothing processed.

I could afford the services because I was not impulse shopping. It was good nutrition and a timesaver. Most of all, it was a gift not having to drag David to the store and supervise him, while trying to think about what to buy with a very conservative budget.

✦ ✦ ✦ ✦ ✦ ✦

David's neurologist took the precautionary step of having David meet with a speech pathologist regarding his swallowing issues. I was glad about this. Like the seizures, the swallowing is a physical manifestation of this disease, and it scares me because it is so real and so observable. You just cannot doubt what you see. In the back of my head, I was thinking that the appointment might be kind of fun. Surely a speech pathologist would have some sophisticated way of figuring out exactly what is preventing David from swallowing. Maybe I would find out what to expect next. Would David start to have trouble swallowing his food?

Once again, David had no idea where he was going; at first, he was a little annoyed. When he saw pretty Julie though, he perked right up. Pretty Julie was very expressive and attentive. She asked him lots of questions and gave him lots of time to answer the questions.

"So, David, sometimes you have a little trouble swallowing the pills?" Julie asks.

"No," David replies. "What? Did I do something bad?"

"No. No, not bad. I think you have had a little trouble with pills, right?" Julie gently prods.

"No. I don't have any trouble. Do I? (turning to me) Do I have trouble?" David asks.

"Yes," I reply. "You have trouble taking your pills, David. You have trouble swallowing them."

"I don't think so," David says in a singsong pshaw tone.

"Well," Julie said. "Let's go get some water and we'll see. Do you want to come with me to get some water, David?" Julie asks David sweetly.

"Oh yes!" David is like a little school boy following his teacher out of the room. He has definitely taken a liking to this lady.

Julie hands David a cup of ice water. David drinks some of it and smacks his lips. "Mmmmm," Julie says. "Mmmmm… Isn't that good?"

"Mmmmm," David replies.

"Now take that pill and pop it in. Just knock it right back. Make it go down," Julie encourages David.

David picks up the pill. I start to cringe. He pops it in his mouth and...*Gulp*. David swallows the pill!

Next pill. A little more water. "Mmmmm," goes David.

"Mmmmm," goes Julie. Pop goes the pill. *GULP*.

To my amazement, David takes the four pills I have brought to the meeting.

Julie assures me that she has seen this before. A different environment, a different person. *Who knows?*

I am shocked. We are invited to come back for another appointment in a week. During the week, I give David half pills and half liquid. He takes all but one pill. One pill gets hidden in a coffee cup in the cupboard, but the rest get swallowed. I give David ice water and say, "Mmmmm."

David says, "Mmmmm." I tell him to pop the pill. He pops the pill and down it goes. More ice water. "Mmmmm," David smacks his lips.

All week I cannot shake the anger I feel as it dawns on me that David has manipulated me this whole time. He has done this for months on end. I have been married to this man for 35 years and, though he may not pass a mental functioning test, he has certainly figured out how to manipulate me. Unbelievable!

Then I think that this may be less conscious manipulation and more a learned behavior. It may be a pattern of stubbornness that he has simply learned how to apply to his advantage. The advantage, of course, is control. There is so little he is able to control, but here is something he can control. He can hold the damn pills in his mouth all night long, and he has done that many times, going to sleep with pills nestled into his cheek. In the morning, he is pulling little pieces of cheek skin out of his mouth where the pills have eroded away the lining of his cheek. Smiling, expressive Julie made him forget the learned behavior. He wanted to please her. After all, she is charming! And I am, well… plainly not charming! Not only that, I'm a nag. So why would he want to please me?

All week, I used Julie's come-hither sweet talk to capture David's attention and get him to swallow the pills and he did. I was the one who needed the teacher. *Thank you, Julie! Where were you six months ago?*

Our follow-up appointment went just as perfectly as the first appointment. Julie told David that he had done so well that she was graduating him. Poor David. He will miss Julie!

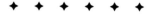

David did seem vulnerable when talking with Julie. He fumbled for words many times, though he was able to get his thoughts across just fine, given her patience with him. Still, he sometimes went from comedy to a sullen frown and grimace trying to think of what he wanted to say, or thinking of something he didn't like. Although he knew we were focusing on pill swallowing, he wanted to tell Julie that he didn't like people taking his things at home. Sometimes what he was saying just did not fit together. His impairments are now so painfully obvious.

So we are indeed into a new phase. Only now, after five years, is there any awareness by people outside our house, our family, our little neighborhood, that something may be wrong with David.

David's ready quick smile and endearing friendliness has always trumped what people might otherwise have wondered about. Who can wonder about a person who takes the time to talk to you and ask how you are doing, to comment on the beautiful weather or say how cute your dog is or how beautiful your baby is?

David is still handsome and winsome. His hair is still mostly dark brown spattered with a little gray at the sides. His eyes are big, greenish brown, and they still sparkle when he talks. It is not the face of illness. We have been ever so normal to everyone else. Few people have known that we both have had our noses level with the ocean water all around us, just barely clearing it so as to keep breathing.

We are still holding hands. We are still together against the world, but the world is getting to be a much more difficult and unforgiving place.

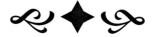

The morning routine before David leaves for the Day Center goes something like this: I have to wake David up about two hours before the van comes to pick him up. I've had to extend the time a bit to make sure that David is seizure-free when he is ready to leave.

I lay out David's clothes on my side of the bed and then shake him or talk to him, telling him it's time to get up. Sometimes he responds quickly and other times he does not. Neither is an accurate forecaster of that morning's seizure activity. While David is still trying to open his eyes, I will go into his bathroom and flush the toilet and I will flush it a few times because David never flushes it. Every woman's nightmare is having a husband who does not flush the toilet or put the seat up to go and down to leave. In David's case, the rim is never up, the misses are near-constant and he never flushes, so it becomes routine for me to go in there, flush it until I can breathe again and then spray it down from top to bottom with a Clorox spray cleaner.

I call to David again as I start to put away the many things that David takes out to touch, hold, set down, move or wonder about. It is usually the little colognes, deodorant, face wash, lotion, and the like from the shelf above his sink. Often he has made an arrangement of towels carefully laid out across the counter with objects placed just so on top. He likes to take apart his electric shaver, for example, and place the pieces all on a towel on the counter, along with his toothbrush and comb and items from the shelves. He can spend hours in the bathroom rearranging his toiletries.

As I call to David again, I move across the room to his dresser and nightstand. There, I usually find a cacophony of CD case tops and bottoms, bare CDs with no cases, a rare few with cases, books pulled out from his nightstand, remnants from his once-full wallet—his Dunkin' Donuts credit card, an old insurance card, some one-dollar bills. The talking doll that he likes, accompanied now by a lady stuffed bear, is set out or sometimes stuffed into a drawer. This represents his work from the evening before. He usually works at this while I make dinner. This work is much less about touching and organization and much more about ownership. He has to see what he owns and know it's still there. When I open the dresser drawers, I pull out what appears to be yesterday's underwear and socks. I thought those already went into the dirty clothes bin, but somehow here they are back in his dresser. It's about ownership and control.

Now David is getting up. I urge him to go to the bathroom as he stands beside the bed, not knowing what to do. He goes and returns. At this point, he may be steady or may already be lurching. I take the time to observe him, particularly his eyes. I've gotten very good at catching him in seizure mode when he cannot focus. Yesterday, he seized and lurched, or lurched and seized, on the way out of the bathroom, crashing first to the floor. When he rose, he then proceeded to crash into the door frame, bruising his knee and bending a finger back as he tried to stop himself. Today, he seems fine. I guide him over to my side of the bed and set him down. There. A shudder. That's a little seizure. No lack of focus today, though. That's good.

"David, let's get dressed," I say.

"What?"

"Let's get dressed, okay?"

"You want a test? A rest? What?"

"No, it's okay. Here, these come off," I say, pointing to his underwear.

"What?"

"These come off."

"Oh."

"Yeah, oh." I start to help him pull them off. Sometimes he throws them at me. I've learned to dodge away and point to the basket on the floor.

I hold his underpants in front of him with the holes lined up at his feet. He takes them from me and turns them around. I take them back and turn them the right way again and help him to put his feet into the holes. He takes my cue and pulls them on.

I tug on his undershirt. "This comes up." Now he is more awake. He pulls the undershirt he has slept in over his head.

I put a clean undershirt over his head.

"Arms," I say.

"What?"

"Arms," I say more forcefully, splaying out an armhole to receive his arm.

He gives me an open hand, which I grab and guide through one armhole. I pick up the other arm from his lap and push it into the other armhole, then pull the undershirt into place.

Next I get his shirt and slide first one arm and then the other into the sleeves. David may try to help button the shirt.

"They make these things so small," David announces. "Why do they make them little like this?" I button his shirt and his sleeves.

I grab his socks and kneel down on the floor. I don't want David to bend over when he is so invariably unsteady in the morning, so I pull his old socks off without asking for his help and wriggle new socks on. I place the shoes in front of his feet. Sometimes I place his toes into the shoes and then rock back on my heels to see what happens.

David just sits there. I wonder if he can feel his toes sitting in the heels of his shoes and wonder why that doesn't compel him to push his feet into them. But it doesn't happen. David just continues to sit there.

"David, shoes," I say. "Shoes." I wiggle a shoe on his foot. He looks down. He starts to push as I continue to wiggle. Somehow we get them on.

I put his glasses on his face. I get his hairbrush and brush down his hair. If he is steady enough, I will invite him into the bathroom to brush his teeth. I put the toothpaste on the brush and hold it in front of him so he can grasp it. Sometimes he wonders what he is supposed to do with it. I point to his mouth. "Brush," I say.

If he is particularly unsteady, I have to leave him sitting on the bed. Then I go and get his morning seizure med right away and bring it back and give it to him. Then I wet and soap up a washcloth and wash and rinse his face while he is still sitting on the bed. His whole body shudders. He doesn't seem to notice. Most often, he makes no comment about the shudders at all. His extra seizure med is having only a minimal effect now. I see less out-of-focus behavior in the morning, but I still see the body jerks. Sometimes they are very minor little shudders, and other times they are violent enough to send him crashing to the floor.

When David is finally steady, dressed, and somewhat groomed, I head him toward the den to sit at the table and have some breakfast. Coffee and juice go in sippy mugs. Sometimes David can be entirely steady up to this point and then all of a sudden, a glass or cup will fly out of his hand, and we have to start dressing all over again.

At this point, my work phone often rings. I answer as though I am at work when, in fact, work couldn't be further from my mind. After David leaves for the Day Center, I can concentrate on work again, not before.

✦ ✦ ✦ ✦ ✦ ✦

It's the 2nd of November, Election Day. Late in the afternoon on this day, I take David with me to the drugstore. We pass one of the election centers along the way where 20 people are lined up and down the road, waving at us with their colorful signs. On a whim, I ask David, "Do you want to go vote?"

"No," David replies. "Not this time. Maybe next one. Then I could go."

I breathe a sigh of relief. What if he had said yes? I voted early in the morning while David was asleep. I stood outside to read the ballot questions because I did not want to take up too much time in the booth. There is just no way that David would be able to understand the ballot. He doesn't even know who is running. How can I tell him who to vote for? It used to be that he had no trouble telling me who I should vote for, pontificating about certain candidates, detailing their positions on the issues, lambasting the opposition, reading the newspaper, listening to CNN and Fox and our local channels. Where is the person who used to do all that?

Later that night, David caught the excitement on TV as the evening news team interviewed candidates and voters alike with their cameras at polling places all over the state.

"I can do that. That's me. I want to...you know. I want. I want. The place you go to. You know. Oh you know. Did you go? I get you went."

Without waiting for me to answer, David continued. "You can't take that away. It's my right. I don't know what you call it. Out? Put? You know."

"Vote? You want to vote?" I ask.

"Yes, that's it. Can you take me? You can't make it stop. I have a right."

"Yes, David, I asked you this morning if you wanted to vote."

"No, you didn't. When did you do that?"

"Earlier today when we were out."

"You never did."

"Look, if you want to vote, I can take you. The polls haven't closed yet."

But now David is angry. It's likely that he knows that he doesn't have the wherewithal to vote, but it comes out as anger directed at me. I have somehow prevented him from exercising his civic duty. It's all my fault. He goes into the kitchen, angrily muttering. I tell him we can go, that it's okay. I don't mind. We can go. He goes to the bedroom, picking up and putting down objects as he passes them. "It's always for you," he says. "All for you. Never for me." This is a familiar theme that David lapses into now.

I have his coat in my hands. "David, let's go."

"No," he replies. "I'm not going. You don't want to let me go. I'm not going."

"Okay, but I offered you the chance to go. I am here to help you go vote if you want to go vote."

Obviously, he just wanted to be angry. He did not really want to go vote. David slammed something down on the dresser and remained angry for the rest of the night.

I don't blame him for feeling angry. I would be angry too. Very angry.

✦ ✦ ✦ ✦ ✦ ✦

We now have a recurring evening routine going. The last two nights are typical. While I am watching TV in the den, David disappears into the bedroom. That would ordinarily be fine, not something I would be concerned about. David has free rein in the house. He goes wherever he wants. Often, it's to his bathroom, the master bath off our bedroom, where he can stand for hours looking in the mirror, touching things, moving things.

Lately, though, he has been doing major sorting, reorganizing, and shifting around of his things. There is really no adequate word to describe exactly what he does. I call it major because it includes completely removing at least one or two drawers from his dresser and nightstand. He then empties out most of the contents onto the bed and relocates his possessions into different drawers. The sorting sometimes looks like a lesson in contrasts rather than similarities. From his nightstand, he takes out his prized feather dusters and puts them into his sock drawer. He moves some of his underwear out of his underwear drawer and puts it in with magazines in the bottom drawer. Belts and CDs are put on top of his dresser and nightstand. Sweatpants are put out on the bed with more CDs, magazines, old papers, and photos.

I notice that he has found the place where I store the many photos waiting to be put into albums. They were in the armoire, but now they have been reorganized into three of his dresser drawers. To make room, he has put a few T-shirts into his nightstand, along with rows and rows of packaged coins from his loose change. The coins have been weighing down drawers for several years now.

When I enter the bedroom, David has a very angry look on his face.

"Why do they do that?" he asks me.

"What?"

Grunt. Groan. "Why? You know. Don't be stupid. You're so stupid. You pretend to be so smart. Oh yes. So. That. It. Wah." Groan again. "You know," he replies.

"Can I help you?" I ask.

"Oh sure. It."

He is struggling with pulling the cuffs of his flannel plaid shirt down to his wrists. The arms of the shirt extend to just below his elbows. Somehow he has put his arms into the sleeves with the shirt inside out, but it is rolled up over his shoulders in such a way that he is being strangled by the shirt holding his arms akimbo.

I go over to him to help him take off the shirt. I explain that it is bedtime, and he does not need to put this shirt on. I pull out a pajama shirt. He jerks away from me.

"Why do I need this? What are you… What?"

"This is your pajama shirt," I say. "It's time for bed." He lets me put it on, but he sees I have brought in his medicine and he balks at that. His face is still contorted in anger.

"No. What? I'm not."

"It's your medicine from your doctor."

"What's that?"

"Medicine."

"What's that?"

"Medicine," I repeat again. "From your doctor. Your doctor says you need to take this to help you."

"That boy. That. He takes my things. They're all. *Tsch.* They're all gone," he says.

"Nobody takes your things," I say. I try to soothe him, but he is not buying it and instead starts to scream at me.

"No! You. You're part of it. You let them. He's your. You think you know. He's your favorite. You let him," he screams. He stands in my face, an inch from my nose.

He starts to unbutton his pajama shirt. I ask what he is doing. He wants to take a shower. It's now 11:30. I am tired and I want to go to bed, but instead I will watch and wait, turn on the shower so he can start, instruct him to wash off the soap, turn off the shower when he is done. Lay a towel on the floor so he does not slip, lay a towel on the sink so he can dry himself off, lay out pajamas on the bed, help him into them.

Sometimes, after all that, he will go off down the hall back to the dark kitchen. I think it's to eat ice cream out of the container because I will often find a spoon on the counter and sometimes I find the remains of the carton in the refrigerator rather than in the freezer. Sometimes he gets into other things, like thinking he has to let the animals in or out. Last night, he left the back slider door wide open all night. I felt the arctic blast when I got up in the morning, but I had been too tired to check things over the night before. What if he had slipped outside in the dark of night? The temps lately have been in the low 30s at night. The nights are destined to become dangerous times if I cannot pay better attention to what is going on.

✦ ✦ ✦ ✦ ✦ ✦

Almost Christmas. Only the briefest of updates now as I struggle to reach back and write, edit, organize so as to put this all into a book that I hope someday will be a major comment on such a devastating disease. There is no way to tell this story retrospectively. I certainly wasn't thinking about a book when I started this. But I am now. I know it will help others. I hope that it's not too sad and too depressing to help others. I hope that it doesn't come across as so much whining and complaining. It's clear that I am making a statement, a plea for more research and a cure. This story, multiplied in homes by the thousands, is the really depressing thought. We have to find a cure.

Last night, David put a T-shirt on his legs once again, with one leg through the neck hole and one leg tightly bound into a sleeve hole, the other sleeve hole hanging loose like an inside-out pocket.

"No, David," I tell him. "Take that off."

"Why," he argues. "Why do you know so much? What's wrong with it?"

"It goes up here on your upper body. It's not for your legs," I try to explain.

"So what. It fits. Why do you think you know everything?"

"Does this make sense to you?"

"Yes."

"How can it? What's this thing hanging here (I point to the hanging sleeve)?"

"That goes there. That's there. Why do you always have to pretend you're so smart?" David remarks, as he gathers the bottom edge of the T-shirt around his waist.

I look at him and wish I had a camera to capture the absurdity of it all. I have no idea why I want to argue with him. He sees something normal. I see it as outrageously nonsensical, but then it hurts no one, so why do I care? Why do I keep trying to fit him into my world? Why do I keep trying to set things right when they cannot be set right? It's pigheaded of me to even think that I can set things back into place. All I am doing these days is making us both miserable.

A few nights ago, I got reflective and wrote this Christmas message to send to those few friends and family we still have:

I particularly like the little quiet time that happens just before Christmas...after concerts, decorating, lights, shopping and going crazy. It's when you finally let yourself think about what to make for Christmas dinner, family, a new year to come and life back to normal.

Well, normal for us is more of the same. But even at that I am so grateful that somehow we have been able to find temporary answers to resolve many of the bumps along the way. I think we realized only recently that David's illness is now readily apparent to others outside the house. Supervision has turned into always keeping him in sight, often with a hand on his arm or holding his hand. Opening doors is sometimes difficult, seat belts impossible. Walking is slow. His meds have been adjusted again, so we are back to an even keel for a while. He continues to attend his Day Center two days a week and I am now bringing in outside help every other week in the evening so I can get out to orchestra rehearsals. Kris and I have been exchanging babysitting and caregiving at other times, and Lisa also helps when she visits from Boston.

Sometimes I wonder how or why this all works out: The fact that David sleeps so late in the morning allowing me to go into the main office twice a week, the fact that I have been able to otherwise work a job mostly from home, the fact that my cello quartet and our teacher agreed to change our weekly practice session to a day when David goes to the Day Center, the friend from David's Coast Guard days who comes on Thursdays to take David out for coffee and once a month takes him up to the base to get a haircut, the personal shopper who now buys my groceries and the fact that it costs me nothing more than what I would have spent on impulse buying if I went myself, the person sent to us from the home-care agency who has turned out to be a genuinely caring person and a good buddy to David, the neighbors who offer to help, our support group members who offer such a wealth of advice and excellent role modeling, the VA medical team that has agreed to take on David's case for monitoring toward eventual long-term care if and when there is room (if and when we are ready), the VA and other dementia and Alzheimer research efforts and those who keep us informed, Elder Services who sent me a Caretaker Appreciation certificate about a week ago when I so needed to be uplifted, David's neurologist who after four years is finally starting to see that he is medically managing an extraordinary person and an extraordinary situation, my commitment made this year to turn my 100+ pages of interesting anecdotal history, meanderings and observations from these past several years into a future publication if I can possibly find the time to devote to writing and editing.

So, what will the new year bring? Hope. Love. Friendship. People to thank again next year at this time!

Hope you have a wonderful Christmas.

Sonja

I do feel ever so lucky, and yet I have these moments when I just have to fight against the invasion and progression of this disease.

David and I continue to walk the neighborhood loop, although David's pace is getting gruesomely slow. Traveling anywhere in the car now takes so much more time. David wanders about the front lawn or the driveway. He either cannot find the car or he cannot understand how to get inside it, so he avoids it altogether. I have to physically place him in the car and close his door before going to my side to get in. He grunts and groans getting in. If he does manage to open the door, he then cannot figure out how to close it.

Every part of our lives is in slow motion. Supervised. Controlled. Deliberate.

Elder Services called to check back with me and suggested that I needed the services of a dementia-experienced RN to help me manage both our home environment and the behaviors I'm seeing. Sounds divine, but it's $200 for a two-hour visit, and my insurance company won't pay for it. *Is this not a necessary medical service? Do I sound like a medically trained professional? Do I have a clue what I'm doing? Why won't you pay for it?* The nurse called and we talked for some time about training caregivers and the lack of that type of support. I laughed when she said it would be a Christmas present for me, but I do believe that. It will be a Christmas present for me.

We had a wonderful Christmas dinner at the Outback with seven friends from our support group. Such a great group of people. I would want to know them for reasons other than illness.

I have now established an extended schedule for the home health aide well into the new year. Kristin will continue to help as well. This will allow me to resume orchestra and quartet for another semester. David balks at having someone in the house who is not family. He complains that he does not need any help. I keep telling him that it's for me. I need the help, and the aide that was sent to us is a very nice young man, very courteous and supportive, neither condescending nor coddling.

The Alzheimer's Services of Cape Cod & the Islands has given me a grant of $500 for "respite care" to help pay for this care. That won't pay for too many home health aide hours, but it's something. It is the first financial help that we have received, so I am ever so grateful. I don't call it respite. I call it my life. It will let me continue to participate in the orchestra for a while longer. With David's all-consuming care, there is little time to practice. At some point, the music that is intended to be a de-stressor in my life will cause me too much stress to continue. For now, I will continue to do what I can.

Year Six

It's the new year and David is progressing along in this disease in his own slow and steady way. I do still take him out, emphasizing how important it is for us to "walk the dog."

In reality, it is so important to walk David. Otherwise, he gets no exercise at all. His slowness is not just evident while we attempt to walk around the block. There's a persistent and pervasive slowness in everything he does, from walking to bending to sitting. He hesitates sometimes when entering a doorway, then steps gingerly through the doorway as though expecting something bad to happen any minute he moves too quickly. After a walk, when we return to the house, David will stand outside the door. I urge him to go ahead, step inside. He does not move. I'm not sure what is going on. Does he not understand that he has to step up? Or, is he not able to direct his foot to step up? Or, is he scared to move at all?

If I come around behind him and put both of my hands lightly under his elbows so as to guide him, rather than push him, then he will respond and step up into the doorway.

Very occasionally, when he slowly raises his sippee cup to his lips, it misses his mouth entirely, taps against his nose, and then he lowers it to his mouth to drink. I have to turn away, walk away, busy myself with something and try not to think about it.

While David does not seem to be in any distress, we have noticed that he huffs and puffs a lot, and he has a wheezing sound in his chest that seems like asthma or an allergy. I know better than to guess at things like this, so of course, I took him to his doctor. I described his condition and noted that he appears to lose his breath at times after walking or just bending over.

His doctor carefully checked him over. His oxygen levels are fine, breathing is fine and lungs are clear. He had a chest x-ray and that was fine too. Nothing wrong. Perhaps an inhaler will help him, and so it was prescribed, but we still don't know why this is happening. It is not purposeful behavior.

There is near constant confusion in the bathroom now. David asks for my help, saying he needs to go to the bathroom. I am grateful when he asks for help because it reduces the antagonisms between us. Yet when I enter the bathroom, he stands there wondering what to do. I remind him that he wants to use the toilet. No, he says he wants to take a shower instead and heads toward the shower.

"Didn't you want to use the toilet?" I ask.

"Oh, yes." David turns back toward the toilet for a few seconds and then turns back to the shower and climbs in with his clothes on. I urge him to come back out and he does, but he also tells me to go away and leave him alone. Later, I find a pee puddle on the carpet.

There's more bowel incontinence. He's not aware of it. I keep my comments to myself and invite him into the bedroom to get changed into something "warmer" so we can go out. He doesn't ask any questions when I change his underwear and wash him down before pulling on a warmer pair of pants.

I wonder about his time at the Day Center, now three days a week. I added Friday mornings so I could expand his supervision and continue to work. We have the home health aide coming on the other two days. David remains cooperative, and so far there have been no problems. There have been changes. They say he is less active; he no longer participates in the chair exercises. When he first started there, he enthusiastically followed the pretty exercise lady, demonstrating arm and upper body exercises. Now, about a year later, he just sits there.

There are good days. David can be very vocal without focusing on his anger and agitation about things. Without the anger, he is able to enunciate his words, pontificating like the old David, remarking about the good guys and the bad guys he sees on the evening news. even if it may not make sense, he is active and engaged, and I encourage him.

There are days when he remarks about the beautiful sunshine, the sparkling snow, the bright blue sky and most of all, the clouds. He loves cloud activity of almost every kind, from scattered foggy drifts to huge and sharply delineated cotton balls. They are all proclaimed "Beautiful!" whether they really are or not. On the subject of clouds, I always boisterously agree with him. I am glad he can see beauty in clouds. When he says "Beautiful!" his whole face breaks into a smile, with his eyes dancing and bright. For just a minute, it seems like the old David is back.

Some days, he slides on his slippers with no problem at all and ambles down the hall from the bedroom. I meet him with a sippee cup of coffee, and I am amazed and happy that this is a good day.

The cold weather brings so many more difficulties getting David dressed and ready to go out. There is no chance of pulling boots onto his feet, so I dress him in sneakers and make sure that the front walk is shoveled bare and salted down. He loves his gloves and demands to wear them, but it is ever so difficult now. When I try to put them on, he splays out his fingers. I close his fingers back up and he splays them out again. Sometimes we laugh. Other times I show my frustration.

Finally, I go out and buy mittens, thinking that will solve the problem. Still, he splays out his fingers so far that I cannot push his hands into the mittens. He is a big man and they don't make mittens large enough for big men with splayed-out hands. More often than not, David goes out to the Day Center van with nothing on his hands. "Don't worry about it," says Henry, the van driver, smiling. "I keep the heat on high!"

Since the third increase in Depakote, I have seen no seizure activity except for the minor jerking movements. These can now occur up to 45 minutes after getting up with no prior occurrence and no warning. I sit with David, helping him with his breakfast, slipping the food back onto the plate or into the bowl when it gets pushed out, making sure that he can grasp and hold his coffee cup. I have every variation of cup and lid. Most of them leak, but at least they prevent coffee from flying all over the room. We are in a stable place.

I must remember to buy an apron for David. What will he think of that?

✦ ✦ ✦ ✦ ✦ ✦

Early in January, I got my Christmas present, which was a two-hour session with the psychiatric nurse who is a specialist in

Alzheimer's Disease. There was nothing she didn't know. After going through his history, Suzanne estimated that David was nine months away from total dependency. I at once thought, *Well, isn't he totally dependent on me now?*

No, she meant that in nine months, David will be totally dependent on me or other people for all activities of daily living including eating, drinking, washing, toileting, walking, moving, communicating. He will not be able to function without 24-hour care and supervision. It was difficult to think about this. Maybe it will be longer for David. Maybe it's not that bad?

He is pretty much maxxed out on his medications. So there will not be any further medical intervention that will be able to help him, she said. His medicines each have a role in speeding along the impulses sent to the brain, but they do not stop the brain cells from continuing to be destroyed. At a certain point, there is nothing left to receive the messages being sent. Everything we do is memory driven, such as going to the bathroom... where it is, where to sit, how to do it, what toilet paper is for. He is losing that memory, and with it the flow of sequencing that forms the necessary components or steps that allow us to complete our daily tasks.

Suzanne explained that his progress in the disease must be measured against child development in reverse (retrogenesis) — independence, reasoning, toileting, using utensils, walking, talking. I should buy Depends now and put them on him. I should watch for injuries, falls, urinary tract infections, pneumonia. All are the most common accompanying serious problems.

I told her about the breathing issues and how cold he seems to be, especially in the morning. Suzanne indicated that it may be a physical reaction of the brain disease in the hypothalamus that may be causing the unusual breathing pattern. That may also explain why he shivers so much at times, usually upon waking up.

I told her that he sometimes cries and that is very hard for me. She said that crying is most likely not an emotional reaction to his losses, but is often biochemically related to the loss of serotonin in the brain, which is necessary to help modulate mood and give us a sense of well-being. He is not sad about what he has lost or can no longer do, because he can't remember what those things were. I can be sad for him about what he has lost, but he is not sad about it. More often he is confused or afraid and is simply looking for reassurance from me.

My responses should be in actions and not words as much as possible. If he is afraid of a light or a reflection, I should go outside and move something or pull the curtain, or put out the light. I shouldn't just say it's okay, it's not a problem, or I'll take care of it. He is 100 percent visual. He cannot think through the words. This hits home big time. I had been aware for some time that I was talking into thin air at times, thinking that I was being a comfort by explaining everything to David. In fact, I was probably further agitating him.

Suzanne said that it's good to engage him in some activities, however minimal. I realized that I had not been doing enough in this regard. Pushing my husband to pursue childlike activities was not high on my priority list. But I realized that I was wrong to think like that. Let him push cards around on the table, Suzanne suggested. Give him silverware to sort. Put photos in a box and tell him they need to be sorted up. Keep his hands very clean. Make an activity out of washing hands…put marbles in the sink. Take the towels out of the bathroom. (David had been using the towels instead of toilet paper.) Develop a routine now to take him to the bathroom at regular intervals. And try again to get the insurance company to understand that we must have help at home.

I asked David's doctor for a "letter of medical necessity" to document David's declining skills and need for supervision. It did not help. Our military insurance, actually a Tufts HMO product, said no way would they pay for any home health aide or home worker. It was out of the question. They would, however, assign a caseworker. Someone would contact me.

I would have to be more vigilant watching out for David. I thought about getting a laptop with a camera on top and placing it in the bedroom to watch over David in the morning. When I am at work in the main office, I can click in over the Internet. That way, if I see that he is waking up, I can rush home to take care of him. At most, I will be a half-hour away. Maybe this will work on the days when I don't have a home health aide.

✦ ✦ ✦ ✦ ✦ ✦

How naive I have been! Our relative calm was short lived. Only a week later, Suzanne's predictions were already coming true. I had left David at home alone, sleeping late as usual, so I could go to work at the main office. Returning home at noon, as was my habit I tentatively opened the side door and peeked around the corner to see if the bedroom door was still closed. It would be a good sign if it was still closed. That meant that he was probably still in bed. This time, however, the bedroom door was wide open, and I sensed that something was very wrong.

I came inside and found David standing in the living room in his pajamas, staring out the front bay window. He turned and started to walk toward me, but it was with a decided limp. He had obviously hurt his foot but kept denying it. He could not tell me what had happened.

His foot was red and very swollen through the center, with toes starting to turn blue. I got him in to see his doctor that afternoon. David was totally oblivious to the injury, feeling no pain at all. He enjoyed seeing his doctor again but had no idea why he was there.

Multiple x-rays later, there was no evidence of a fracture, but fractures don't always show up right away, and they don't always show up on x-rays. The next day, Kristin came over to take a look and immediately said, "Oh Mom, that's definitely broken. That's a broken foot. I've seen plenty and there's no question." She got back on the phone with the doctor the next day. A few days later, a visit to an orthopedic specialist and an MRI proved her right. David had three fractures across the top of his foot.

I pieced together what had happened from the appearance of the bedclothes on David's side of the bed and the dresser, which was at an odd angle. David got up without me there to help. He had a seizure, and as he fell to the floor, his foot slid under the front bottom edge of the dresser. I found bruises on the back of his neck where his neck had struck the footboard of the bed as he fell. It all made sense. Needless to say, I felt terrible for leaving him alone.

He is now in a large plastic boot from his foot to his knee. It further complicates getting him dressed and undressed each day. His jeans won't fit, so I have him in running pants with wide or zippered legs. Surprisingly, he is learning how to lumber through the house with his gimp leg, and, thankfully, he does not blame me for what happened.

✦ ✦ ✦ ✦ ✦ ✦

David is now sundowning, as they say. I hate to use a book term to describe him. The book version of sundowning and David's version are not exactly the same. He is not just more irritable and uncooperative in the late afternoon and early evenings, he seems astoundingly unable to comprehend himself and his surroundings at this time of day. Maybe it is partly due to changes in medications. His Paxil, which was up to 60 milligrams a day to control his aggression and moodiness, is now back to 40 milligrams a day. I don't even remember why. David is certainly less angry now, more complacent. Maybe the doctor thought he did not need as much, maybe it would help with his bowel incontinence. But then we have these late afternoons from another planet.

It's a Catch-22; the late afternoon is the same time of the day when he tends to need to have a bowel movement, only he no longer recognizes it as a normal bodily function. It is something distressing. He says he must be sick and shouldn't he go to the doctor? Suddenly it overcomes him and he races to the bathroom, dragging and bumping the boot down the hall. When he gets there, he cannot figure out how to negotiate the toilet fast enough.

He seems to experience more delusions late in the day. There are "waves" on the bed. David remarks how crazy it is to have all these waves all over the bed. He tries to pat them down and make them go away. Validating this perception is very difficult for me. It feels deceptive. Not because I am such a purveyor of truth and honesty, but because it is diminishing to David and damaging to our relationship. So, I tell him that it must have been the cat who pushed the covers around and made all those bumps or waves on the bed. He is now convinced that we have 50 kittens who sleep under the covers! He pushes them out of the way to get into bed. He thinks it's funny. I think it's sad. He sees reflections in the TV or on the glass of our windows that seem to be in strong colors. "Oh look. Look!" he will remark in amazement and wonder. I'm sure he thinks I'm blind as a bat because I can't see the colors.

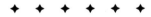

I had a late meeting yesterday, so David spent most of the day with his caregiver. They were out in the back yard when I got home, walking around, enjoying the unusually warm winter day. The dog played happily at their feet. When the caregiver left for the day, David stayed in the back yard while I headed to the bedroom to get changed. He seemed content to be out there.

I returned to the den a few minutes later and opened the slider to tell David to come in. As he did so, he matter-of-factly told me that he was "all dirty." I thought that he was commenting about his shoes and looked down. Not exactly. He told me he had just pooped outside because I was not there to help him.

Like a crazy person myself, I asked him, "What do you mean you pooped outside?"

"Right there. Right there. I pooped right there. It's your fault."

I looked outside in the grass where he was pointing. There was a pile of poop in the grass like a St. Bernard's.

"You've got to be kidding!" I exclaim to David. "You can't just go out there and poop like a dog!"

"It's your fault," David repeats.

Okay, so this is absurd. Is he now controlling his dependence on me, to the extent that he expects my immediate help and when it is not available, he will damn well poop on the lawn to pay me back for not being right there?

"David. David. You can't do this," I say again.

"Why not?" David argues back. "Everyone does it."

"No, they don't. Dogs do it. People don't do it."

"Yes, they do."

"No, they don't." I have to stop arguing. David needs to be changed. He has poop on his legs and his pants and under one shoe. There is a smear on the carpet.

✦ ✦ ✦ ✦ ✦ ✦

The boot is surely causing some of this bathroom confusion. It seems that all of a sudden, David is having real problems negotiating the distance to the toilet seat. He thinks the seat is much lower than it really is. He thinks he is falling, and is it possible? He seems scared and frightened of using the toilet. No wonder he pooped outside. It was the lesser of two evils.

I try to stay vigilant for when David needs to go to the bathroom and follow him. Sometimes I am too slow and I find him standing up, pants down, in the process. Towels all around smeared brown. He puts poop on the sink, runs the water and expects it to go down.

When I do manage to time things just right so that we are both in the bathroom together, David fights against me. I try to help lower him to the toilet, but he pushes back up and cries out as though I am hurting him. The meds have now caused his weight to hover at about 240 pounds. It's an increase of 60 pounds and I literally cannot handle him myself. Add the fact that he is fighting against me and it becomes an impossible situation. We fail miserably. David wonders what on earth I am trying to do as I steadily talk to him about how we need to get him situated. There I go talking to him too much. I can't seem to stop. Why do I think that I can get him to understand by using words?

Meanwhile, the urge to go overcomes him to such a degree that he is in a world of panic, pain and discomfort.

I hate this. He hates this.

Yesterday I bought Depends size extra large, bed pads, flat heavy rugs for the bathroom floor and a rolling table with a wheel base that can slide under a chair or a bed so the table top can be brought up close. I need more elastic-waist pants for David. I need a rubber rug that can lie over the carpet near the bed. I need more pajamas and I need all the baby wipes the drugstore has on hand. Not only that, I need someone to go to the store for me to get all this stuff!

While the Depends are ever at the ready, I have only ever slipped them on David at night. I have not yet started to put them on him during the day. So far, he has not noticed what I put on him. I am glad. I thought he would chastise me for making him look like a baby. If I put them on him during the day, someone at his Day Center will notice and David will get embarrassed. Worse, the Day Center will say that if he is no longer continent, he can no longer attend. That would be such a loss for David and such a loss for me. It's like walking a tightrope trying to decide the best thing to do each day.

I have started to mark certain towels with a big black X. That means that they have been used in the bathroom and on the floor. I soak them in bleach and reuse them for the same purposes. When utterly exhausted, I throw out dirty underwear and pants and just go out and buy more.

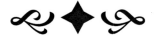

Quite apart from the negative toileting experiences, we have achieved a certain milestone together where I do think that David more frequently recognizes some of his dependence on me and waits patiently for my help. He is less bitter and antagonistic towards me.

I enjoy making our lunches and sitting down with him to eat together. It often occurs to me that this is how it might have been in the future, and we are playing out future scenes that will never occur. In our future retirement together, we would both be enjoying our respective retirements, our independence from the rat race. We would have time to sit together at home, to play cards or watch a movie, to take a walk together. The only difference would be that we would be in our 70s or 80s, not our 50s.

I feel strongly how much we need to acknowledge this special time together. It seems particularly enhanced by the recent snowy winter weather. I make soup and grilled cheese sandwiches. We watch the snow pile up at the back door.

There are still good days. David will get up and seem to be in a good mood. I give him a shower. He stays in a good mood, eating his sandwiches, watching a little TV with me. He tries to clear the dishes, but really can't manage more than a glass and a spoon. Still, we work together to get the dishes to the sink. Then he gets tired. He needs to go back to bed. And so I lead him back to the bed where I have him sit, while I take off the damnable boot. He lies down and goes to sleep. A young man, already old. I close the door.

Sometimes I give myself permission to wallow in the combined grief and wonder that I find myself in. I watch my life swim around in front of me, thinking about how difficult this is getting. How will we manage? How will I manage? David's beginning toileting confusion has now become ultra aggravated as a result of this injury and having to drag a heavy boot around on one foot. His heavy breathing has increased. His fatigue is so apparent. Yet even through the worst of times, he frequently regains his good personality, laughing and talking again. His eyes sparkle as he laughs. Those sparkling laughing eyes. It's something this illness cannot take away from him.

✦ ✦ ✦ ✦ ✦ ✦

A few days ago, I woke up with a start to find David standing in the bathroom in his pajamas, just standing there. I said, "Are you okay? Is everything okay?"

He responded, "It's so weird."

"What's weird?" I asked.

"It's so weird," he repeated. Then he walked back into the bedroom and after three steps suddenly dropped like a load of bricks to the floor. His back hit the corner of the nightstand as he crumpled into the small space between the night table and the doorway to the bathroom. His face was collapsed into such a mixture of sadness, anger and exasperation. I helped him up and he was able to stand up, but that was it. He could not follow my instructions to move to the bed, to turn, to take a step. He was frozen and unresponsive for a minute or two, then he allowed me to guide him to the side of the bed. Sitting there with his head down, he continued to be unresponsive to me for two to three more minutes. I was then able to finally coax him into lying back down and extending his legs under the blankets.

This crumpling to the floor is so unbelievably sudden. It's no wonder that he has already had a serious injury with a broken foot. *Here we go again. And how many days has it been since the nurse warned me to beware of injuries? I hate this.*

I am beyond disillusioned, as I am now thrust into a world of providing 24-hour care for David. Of course, I knew this would happen at some point, but I did not think it would be so soon. It means that I am now tied down 24/7, and relief costs me at least $21 an hour. I don't make $21 an hour. My insurance company won't help. In fact, even though David's doctor prescribed the help, the local visiting nurse association turned us down flat. They said that if David is able to go out to a Day Center two or three times a week, then he did not qualify for at-home care.

I met with a social worker who explained that there is something called being "psychologically home bound." That means that the person could not possibly go out on his or her own, in a car or walking or in any form whatsoever. They are 100 percent dependent on someone else to arrange to take them out and to provide transportation. *Well, isn't it obvious that David is psychologically home bound? Isn't it obvious that he is a person with a medical condition who needs medical care in his home?*

I got nowhere with our insurance company.

I did step up the hours I was getting from the home health agency, at my expense of course. At the same time, I got a call back that our current aide was no longer working, and so we would be getting a new person. This was something I had not considered, that the agency I was using could, at will, change who they were sending over.

At first, I was aghast at the thought of having to convince David all over again that there was a good reason why someone he did not know should be in our house watching over him. I had worked so hard to get David to be accepting of the person we already had. Even so, he would scowl and complain at times.

Luckily, Jack was assigned to us and Jack turned out to be a gem. It's been several weeks now and Jack is genuinely pleased to help take care of David. And in fact, he has volunteered to help me out with so many things, including the lawn mowing and fertilizing.

Jack enjoys making lunch for David, has no problem getting him in and out of the shower, and now regularly takes him on outings for lunch or coffee. Jack volunteers at a local senior center at lunchtime and has brought David along with him several times. Soon David became the star guest, socializing with everyone, especially the ladies. David certainly enjoys these outings. So, when I thought that it couldn't get any worse, suddenly everything is feeling much better.

✦ ✦ ✦ ✦ ✦ ✦

It's February now and we have Jack coming on a regular schedule. I am finding it helpful that Jack is very observant of any changes in David, and he seems to take everything in stride. David's minor body jerking continues, but it has not been a problem. There is some shaking in David's hands that wasn't there before. It's as though he is developing a kind of palsy. He is also starting to have difficulty sitting down at times, feeling for the empty space behind him, unsure if there is a chair to sit on, obviously experiencing growing spatial orientation problems.

When Jack leaves for the day and I retreat to my desk in the basement, David can be counted on to go on eating binges in the kitchen, so I have to continue to be careful about leaving food out or in easy reach in the cupboards. Nothing I can do about the ice cream, nor do I necessarily want to do anything about the ice cream. That's the last thing I would ever want to take away from David. So, I stock up extra half gallons in the freezer to replace the ones that are left out on the counter or parked in the refrigerator alongside the milk and orange juice.

Bernie continues to visit weekly. He'll sit in the den telling David all about his family, updating him on the news and the Coast Guard. When it's time to take David up to the base to get a monthly haircut, Bernie helps to get him ready. In one of David's pockets, Bernie puts the 10-dollar bill I hand to him. He tells David, "Here you go. Now that is for the lady who is going to cut your hair. You want to give her a ten-dollar bill, because that includes the tip. That makes it easy." In another pocket, he puts David's military ID card. "Here you go, buddy. That's in case they stop us at the gate and they want to know who you are. I'll tell them who you are. Career Coastie. That's who. But this is just in case." He puts David's Dunkin' Donuts credit card in yet another pocket. "This is for when we go get coffee. Now hold on to that." If I was taking David out, I would have put all these things in my purse, trusting David to take care of nothing at all. I treat David like a patient. Bernie still treats him like a friend.

One afternoon after getting coffee, Bernie brought David home and didn't say a word but brought David into the kitchen. David had peed in his pants and was all wet. I told David that we needed to go get changed and he obediently walked with me to the bedroom. Afterwards, I brought him into the den and sat him down in his favorite chair. Bernie was there waiting for him. I thought about the cloth seats Bernie had in his car. Still, he did not say a word and he was back the next week, ready to take David out again.

A neighbor came over late one night and helped us shovel out after a snowstorm. David and I were out there making little progress. I wanted David to help shovel out the heavy area at the end of the driveway, but he wanted to brush off the cars instead. Maybe I was a little loud telling him he needed to listen to me. Maybe my frustration showed. In any case, a neighbor showed up to help.

I am ever so grateful for these people who seem to float like shadows in and out of our lives, just when I need them most.

✦ ✦ ✦ ✦ ✦ ✦

We are having very difficult cleanliness issues in the bathroom and sometimes in the rest of the house. David is using towels to wipe himself and, even then, doesn't do a very good job.

I try instructing him. It's useless. He looks at me as though he absolutely hates me. I am not only in his personal space, I have invaded his personal space in every possible way. He resents me. I resent that he resents me. I follow him around because I don't trust him to take care of himself. He will come out of the bathroom with dirty hands and fingernails and proceed to the kitchen, pull out a dish and start to get the ice cream out of the refrigerator. I run screaming at him to stop. It's getting ludicrous.

When I get to David in time to help him, it is a painstaking process to remove his boot, undress him and get him situated quickly enough to avoid disaster. I put towels around him by force of habit now so that he does not slip and fall on a wet floor. Sometimes we have to go from the toilet directly into the shower, and I have to use all of my diplomatic skills to convince him that this is necessary.

Whatever I was trying to accomplish at the time has to be set aside for later. I get David clean and warm and comfortable again. Cleaning the bathroom and his clothes will have to wait while I fix dinner and try to get in another few hours of work before the end of the day. I am cleaning until midnight, then up at 5:00 a.m. to start work.

✦ ✦ ✦ ✦ ✦ ✦

Still February and I am reaching the end of my rope. Feeling so depressed. My life is so meaningless at this point. I feel lost and left behind, and I have a growing and extreme need to know *how long will this last*? I cannot do this for another five years. Is that a possibility? Could he really go on and on and on like this for maybe another five years? I am not sure that I can do this for another five minutes. This is a life really not worth living…for either of us.

How do I rise above it when I find him red-faced and panting in the bathroom, holding a sock covered in poop, with more on the counter, in the sink, on his underwear and pants, on the floor, on the bedspread. Instead of being glad that I am there to help him and instead of welcoming my help, he drops his jaw and wags his finger a quarter-inch from my nose and scowls at me, saying in his mumbo-jumbo lingo, "This is you. Your your fall it…your fault. All you! You think you're so impor… important. You did this to me. It's you. You feed me. Look. Look. Look what you do to your own husband. You think you know you…you you you awful excuse for a wife."

Then he slams the door in my face. The room reeks. I turn on the ceiling fan and open the window and walk away. I guess I am an awful excuse for a wife. He is screaming our reality back at me.

I look somewhere deep within me to find the energy to make my way back and push open the door, only to have it slammed in my face repeatedly. I bring plastic bags and tell him to drop the sock in, drop the underwear in. He refuses and refuses, then finally he does it. I gingerly pick up other things and drop them in. I can't reach beyond him to get the plastic gloves that are on the shelf in the bathroom. I think I am going to be sick.

Again he is telling me in garbled speak what a rotten person I am, how I only do things for myself, how I have poisoned him. As I try to ease my way around him, he is lunging at me with his angry accusations. I tell him to move back. He won't do it, but I have managed to get past him to turn on the shower. Now he tells me that I have broken everything because I am so stupid. The shower doesn't work because I am stupid. I turn the faucet until the water runs warm and tell him to get in. He refuses and refuses, standing there with stuff all down his legs, taking an angry stance against me.

I squeeze past him to the freedom of the doorway. Again I think I am going to get sick. Again I tell him to get in the shower. He backs in, slowly, while staring angrily at me, staring right through me.

I slip out of the bathroom and bring the plastic bag of clothes to the washing machine where I soak them, thinking as I go that I am in desperate need of a diaper pail. How can I get organized enough to get in the car and go to the drugstore to get one? I can't. I can't leave David to get the diaper pail. Not only that, I left him in the shower upstairs. I can't do that. I have to get back there. *What am I doing? I'm going crazy.*

After David is put to bed in clean pajamas, I sit down and stare at the TV. I don't want to go to bed. There is no joy in sleep. I don't know what bed to get in. I can't sleep in the room that still smells so bad. That's my half of a bed in there, but it's certainly not appealing. I don't want to sleep in the other bedroom. I don't want to watch TV. I don't want to do anything, in fact, except sit and stare straight ahead of me. I'm awake staring straight ahead and then I'm asleep. When I wake up, I'm still staring straight ahead. I can't move.

Is this what it feels like to have a breakdown? Am I really losing it or am I just feeling sorry for myself in an extreme kind of way? I lie down on the bed in the other bedroom and fall asleep, but then I'm awake again. I get up and go down to the office and do three hours of work. Why? It's 4:00 a.m. on Saturday. Then I watch a movie.

Somehow I get through the night. Now it's time to get David up again. To deal with him again. I don't want to look at him. I don't want to talk to him. I don't want to live this life anymore, but there is no other life that I want to live. What to do? What to do?

I get David up around noon, give him his medicine, get him dressed. I make soup and sandwiches and coffee and cake for lunch. As I serve it to him, he says, "So, did you have a nice time?" in such a mean and sarcastic tone. "What have you been doing all this time anyway? More fun?" He knows I'm a mess and he knows he is hurling daggers at me. I swear he knows it. His tone is scornful and demeaning and critical. It's as though he has been so degraded by his lack of physical control and his dependence on me that he is striking out in any way that he can.

At the same time, I am sinking lower and lower and lower. I think this job is for someone else, not for me. I can't feel abused and be a good caregiver. He will be better with someone else whose buttons can't be pushed as easily as he can push mine. He will be spending a lot more time alone until I can get him cared for by someone else.

✦　✦　✦　✦　✦　✦

Of course, my threats serve only to momentarily let me feel better. I am so shocked at how permeable my spirit has become that I can so easily allow misery to invade every cell of my being like that, to get to such a low point. A lot of it is due to fatigue. The days are bad enough, but then so are the nights. I have to keep one eye open watching for David trying to get up on his own. I can feel it when his weight leaves the bed and I fight to open my eyes and fling myself out the other side of the bed to race to wherever he is. The constant vigil causes constant anxiety.

It's not always bad. Some days, David seems able to go to the bathroom and takes care of himself reasonably well. Then we have days that are sort of in between. David seems fine, but then I find dirty wipes pushed into the pocket of his pants and I realize that I should have been watching over him more closely. Then we have the disaster days when David's physical control is totally absent, his anger and my anger are like twin fusions, and we find so many unnecessary ways to make each other miserable. There are not enough good days to reclaim some measure of our marriage and our love for each other. We are too busy either fighting the disease or fighting each other.

We are still pending our second VA appointment. It has been rescheduled twice. I found out that we will no longer be seeing a doctor with the program. Our appointments from now on will be with the nurse practitioner. I'm sure they have too many patients and too few doctors, so I can't be upset about this. Besides, I was quite impressed with the nurse practitioner assigned to our case.

Only now, they tell me that they are scheduling us with someone entirely different whom we have not met before. Why? I have called and left a message that we are having problems, and we need the other nurse practitioner who knows exactly where David is in this disease. We cannot waste time on a reassessment. The social worker agrees, but no one calls me back. Still waiting and waiting.

Finally, I get the appointment rescheduled yet again, and this time with the same nurse practitioner. The social worker tells me not to worry, that waiting for an appointment and seeing someone different will not jeopardize David's eligibility for long-term care, but I am starting to worry anyway. *What if the staff changes and the person who originally promised David a place in their program is no longer there? What if there is simply no room in the program for David once he is determined ready?* The VA Alzheimer's units are just not that big. No one graduates. We would be waiting for someone to die, as morbid as that sounds, and given how fast David's condition has progressed, can I really depend on the VA hospital to have a bed available right when David needs it? I am getting pretty good at advocating for what we need, but there is just not a lot out there in the way of resources.

I have set a goal to visit some of the local nursing homes who take Alzheimer's patients and who also take Medicaid. Our backup plan will have to be that I will pay directly for long-term care until we run down our assets to the level at which we can apply for Medicaid.

I hate the thought of having to apply for Medicaid, but the cost of a nursing home is running at least $9,000 a month, and our insurance won't cover it. I have been to two attorneys for advice already. David's military pay and his small municipal disability pension will be applied to his nursing home bill. Without his income, I won't be able to pay for the mortgage and other bills on my own, at least not with what my current job pays. David's truck, our cash assets plus my retirement savings will be considered joint assets that will have to be reported and potentially turned over to help pay for his care.

I am particularly incensed that the government would come after my retirement savings. Why impoverish me? I can accept having to look for a better job. I can accept selling the house and reducing my expenses. The caregiver gets a bum deal, for sure. After everything that I have already given up, how is it fair for them to take part of my retirement savings, particularly when they will have already taken all of David's retirement income?

These are some of the thoughts running through my head that keep me up at night.

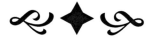

We had our second visit to the VA hospital. We were met by the same nurse practitioner and social worker whom we had seen on our previous visit. Both were very understanding. David sat in the waiting room for the most part with his boot on, periodically thumping down the hall to look for the bathroom.

I explained what we had been dealing with over the past six months, including the beginning bowel incontinence, continued seizure issues and, most recently, his fall and injury. This time, they spent more time asking me about how I was dealing with it all, how I was keeping up. They wanted to know what I was doing to take care of myself. I explained that I now had more help, with a caregiver coming in a few times a week, and David was still going to his day program. Without this help, I wasn't sure how I would have been able to cope. So many new things to worry about. As we drove up to this appointment, David's hands seemed to be all over the car. He kept touching the door handle and then the gearshift. He even reached over to grasp the keys in the ignition, all while I was driving down the highway. Everything he did, every movement, needed monitoring.

The next appointment was scheduled for four months out, but they counseled me that, if necessary, I could call and let them know that it was getting very difficult, perhaps too difficult. They encouraged me to call.

Going home, it was a two-hour drive from hell to watch the traffic with one eye and David's hands with the other. Toward the end, it was clear that David had had enough. I had him strapped in tightly, but he started adjusting his whole body in the seat as though he was going to open the door and step out onto the highway. I had to stop for half an hour to give him a break. It seemed to take forever to get home that day.

✦ ✦ ✦ ✦ ✦ ✦

It's the end of March, and I am finding it difficult to continue to write when I just don't have anything positive to say. Instead, I have a low, bad feeling most of the time.

A friend from our support group is looking to place her husband into long-term care soon. He will probably need it before David will. He is about David's age, and at this point, he is up all night taking very aggressive stances, such that she and her children have to lock themselves into their bedrooms at night to stay safe. What kind of crazy balancing act is this when family members have to be nurses and policemen? Like me, she has limited resources, but she is reaching maximum overload fast.

So we went together to visit a few of the local nursing homes able to take Alzheimer's patients. The experience made us both cry. Everyone is 80 or 90 years old in these places! These are the wrong places for our husbands! Not only that, the cost is exorbitant. We are untrained caregivers working for free because we just don't have the choice to opt out. They are the professionals, but they charge $300 a day. Our insurance companies won't pay either way—either for at-home care or for long-term care at a nursing home. So I guess everyone is happy with this arrangement of letting untrained spouses carry the burden until they fall apart or die themselves. This is a no-win situation, especially for the Alzheimer's patient.

I learned that the state has two state-supported care facilities for veterans. They are not part of the federal Veterans Administration. How did I miss this before? The one closest to us is in Chelsea, just north of Boston. It's called the Chelsea Soldiers' Home. I worked all night one night filling out an application for David. They only have 18 beds in their Alzheimer's wing, but who knows? Perhaps it will be another place I can add to my defense lineup.

I had a meeting with a local health-care representative at one of the Senior Centers. He was so anxious to try to help me, and yet, what help could he offer? None. As I went through my options, his advice was to not quit my job. That was one of my options. I figure that I can last about two years taking care of David by myself at home 100 percent of the time if I give up working entirely. The only bill I really have to worry about is the phone bill. I will need to be able to call 911. Other than that, I really don't care anymore.

"No," he said. "Don't quit your job. That's the last thing you want to do. Your job is your only connection to other people and the rest of your life." I had to think about that. He was right. I had become a hermit taking care of David. There were no other people in my life except people at work and people I played with in the community orchestra. I had already decided that this would have to be my last season with the orchestra, so that will leave work as my only connection to anyone in the outside world. I could not contemplate "the rest of my life," but I knew I didn't want to be isolated.

Another option was to ask Jack to move in with us. I could give him the rooms in the basement. When we first moved into the house, I thought that I would use these rooms for David's caregiver some day. Is that day here? It seems so foreign. What would Jack think about this?

✦ ✦ ✦ ✦ ✦ ✦

I had kept in touch with David's older sister in Texas periodically. It was time to call her. I tried to explain to her, without alarming her unnecessarily, that David was entering the final stages of Alzheimer's Disease. I told her that he was still able to communicate, but soon he would not be able to do so. She understood immediately and arranged to come for a visit in April.

David recognized her right away and smiled broadly. Carlann engaged him for hours in back-and-forth table talks about their family and how they had spent their childhoods in delicious mischievousness. It did not matter to her that it took David so very long to respond or ask a question. After all, she was there to spend time with him.

"Where is...Mom?"

"She's gone, David," Carlann gently replied.

"Where is...Charlie?"

"He's gone too, David. But I'm here. I came all the way from Texas. I'm here."

David's mood brightened considerably, as did mine. A visit from Carlann was just what we both needed. Kristin and Lisa came over. We had family dinners at home and we also took Carlann out for a Cape Cod dinner of fish and chips. She and David visited his favorite coffee place several times.

Carlann told me how grateful she was that I was taking such good care of David and that whatever I decided about his care, well, she was 100 percent behind me. It meant so much to me to hear that.

✦ ✦ ✦ ✦ ✦ ✦

David has been having more significant seizure activity, and he has also started to have more episodes of loose stools and diarrhea. Both are causing me no end of anxiety and frustration. I look at him as he sits in the chair in the bedroom. He seems happy and content, all dressed in clean clothes, his face nicely washed, his hair brushed, his teeth brushed, his glasses cleaned. I have not washed my own face in two days, and I am wearing yesterday's clothes. Still, I'm proud of my work. I do take good care of him.

We had a visit from a nurse from the Chelsea Soldiers' Home. Much to my surprise, she came to us to do an assessment. I thought she would be examining David, but instead, she mostly examined me, asking me question after question, each time nodding as I replied, describing some of David's more recent issues.

He has a sore shoulder that has been x-rayed. He winces and cries out in pain when I try to dress him. I can't figure out when he injured it, but there have been so many times that he has fallen to the floor in a seizure drop that I have lost track. Nothing is broken, but he is now scheduled for physical therapy three times a week, and so I have to take him there. I am unsure if it is a good idea. *If I don't take him to physical therapy, will someone think that I am not doing the right thing, not taking care of him? Do they have any concept of what it takes to get him ready to go out, to put him in the car, to walk him into the building?*

I tell the nurse that there is a restlessness in David that is becoming more pronounced. He literally prowls through the house looking for trouble, taking things apart, pulling things off the counters, ransacking the kitchen to find and eat whatever food is accessible.

His lack of awareness when he has a bowel movement and his lack of understanding when it comes to cleaning up still amaze me. Maybe it's because David finds more and more ways to aggravate me. Of course I'm being unreasonable. David is not trying to aggravate me, but when I find dirty brown wipes on the kitchen counter, I want to scream! When I find poop in the kitchen sink, I marvel at how he is able to actually walk around the house secretly holding it, and I do not realize what's going on!

I tell the nurse that I am not able to keep up. I just can't keep up. That was before the episodes of diarrhea started. Now what will I do? She nods her head.

I also tell her that I have had it with the lack of seizure control. We are not even close to really helping David with this. Standing in the kitchen one day, I happened to read all of the small print right to the end that accompanied David's refill of Aricept. Seizures are a very rare but possible side effect. I decide on my own to reduce his Aricept slowly. *Will I get into trouble for this?* Part of me worries and part of me announces that I really don't care. I am the one who is caring for David and no one else wants to be in charge, so I am in charge. It's worth a try. So far, after a small decrease, it seems to me that his morning tremors are not as bad as they were last week.

Why do even nice things turn out to be problems? Along with hats and belts and shirts, David has been taking off his glasses repeatedly. I find them on the counter, on the table, on the floor. I put them back on him and he takes them off. Jack didn't know and bought him a pair of nice new sunglasses. He looked cool for about a day, but that's about how long it took before he lost them.

Last night, he took off his glasses and used them to eat his dinner. He actually scooped his food onto the lenses of his glasses and licked them clean, never once realizing what he was doing.

Reflections seem to be driving him nutty. He sees them all around now: in the TV, in the windows, in the glass of the microwave and the slider. He points to the floor to something invisible and seems to be watching it move.

One day this week when I woke David up, he looked at me in the strangest way. I asked, "Do you know who I am?"

He stammered back, "You are…are…my…w…wife."

"Good, David. What is my name?"

He could not tell me. I told him, "My name is Sonja."

His reply? "Good guess."

The nurse closed up her notebook. As she headed for the door, she turned to me and said, "I'm going back to find him a bed. I don't know how long it will be. But I will find him a bed. You need your life back."

✦ ✦ ✦ ✦ ✦ ✦

More and more often now when I look at David, I feel that pang of alarm in my chest or stomach. It's a danger signal. A back-off signal, only I can't back off. I am the caregiver. It's also very much like the feeling you have after a really close call while driving, when you are swelled up and tense and not quite believing that you just avoided an accident. The feeling you have before relief floods in. Only there is no relief for us in our situation. It is just danger, danger, danger all the way, and we cannot get out of the way. We are the deer in the headlights.

There is a visual thing going on. He cannot pick up the nuts I give him to eat, and it's not because he can't see them. They seem to move from where he thinks they are.

When walking, he lifts up his leg to step over cracks in the sidewalk and does something with his hands, pulling at his fingers repeatedly, grasping at something invisible. Sometimes I hold a cup of juice out in front of his face, asking if he wants a drink. He can't see the juice. He is looking far beyond the juice at something I cannot know about. He is already there. Someplace else.

He comments about things quite often, but his sentences are jagged and without subject or object. If you say something to him, he responds with words that bear no relation to what you just said.

There is nothing for him to do except to get into trouble, breaking a dish, pouring soap on the counter, binging on half a cake while I try to work, running the water and walking away, carrying objects from one location to another, putting my keys in his pocket. I tried giving him boxes of pictures to look at and sort. I tried giving him a box of silverware to help sort out. These things did not attract his attention for more than a minute.

David is now more frequently peeing on the bathroom floor and wetting his pants at the Day Center when he can't get to the toilet in time. They have been very good to him there, but they also indicated that mealtimes have become difficult, as he now requires one-on-one assistance. He can no longer grasp and hold a cup. Sometimes he can handle a fork or spoon, other times he just uses his fingers.

When David arrives home from the Day Center today, he is in distress, needing to get to the bathroom. He just can't make it all the way down the hall. It's happened so many times and it's pathetic to see—pathetic to watch him try to maintain himself as normally as possible when out of the house, only to have these awful attacks as soon as he enters the doorway. I call the Center to thank them sincerely for their wonderful care and attention. David will not be returning.

✦ ✦ ✦ ✦ ✦ ✦

We visited a different day care center this week. This one is medically supervised with a nursing staff on hand. David felt very much at home there. They were reassuring and David was very relaxed. Hopefully he will start to go there two days a week, but we have to wait for an opening. The director said there will be at least one day a week available soon, but otherwise the program is full right now. It's a step up in care and very expensive, but they will be able to handle the incontinence. If David attends this program at least a few days a week, and if I continue to have an attendant come to take care of David at our house for another few mornings or afternoons during the week, then I think we can make it until I can get David into long-term care. I realize that it's a healthy admission on my part that I must have this help from others. There is really no choice. As for the expense, I really don't care anymore.

I don't care about a lot of things anymore. Mostly I feel like an idiot trying to do the normal things. Making dinner, washing dishes, putting some bulbs in the ground, washing down the patio set. I wonder why. *Why am I doing these things? None of it matters. It won't change anything. I'm tired and sad. Why do I keep trying to do things that make me more tired? Can I be any sadder?*

✦ ✦ ✦ ✦ ✦ ✦

It is 16 days before David's 58th birthday, and this is my last entry. Beyond this point, I will not go because David is now held physically as well as mentally captive by this illness. We are in a sad and empty goodbye place, and there just is no more sharing to be done with others. I have to focus on David now and the time that we have left together. There is nothing that I can do to stop this. I have no idea if I have offered David any comfort along the way. So much has been about me and not him. I do realize that. It doesn't mean that I don't love him. I love him with all my heart and soul.

I will continue to support David's ever-changing world of normal for as long as I can. Then, I will turn him over to others who are more experienced than I am and more patient than I am. I feel secure knowing that his mostly good-natured personality will protect him and provide him with the care and support he needs and deserves. I know I will find the right place for him, whether it's the VA hospital or a local nursing home. I've met many good people, and I know David will find comfort and security in eventual round-the-clock care. It is odd to me how very obvious this all seems to me now. The fact that I would feel reassured by placing David in long-term care seems crazy, given that so many months ago, it was something that I could not really wrap my head around.

It's been long and difficult. I know I have done some things well and other things not so well. I haven't liked having to figure things out for myself, mostly by myself. That has made this a very lonely journey. I am grateful, of course, for the help from time to time that we have received. I am also grateful for the truly nurturing caregivers, social workers and others whom I tried to learn from and emulate.

Sick people don't exist in a bubble. There are relationships that continue to evolve each and every day. There is a present and future impact on other people. It has been a cruel thing to watch my partner in this life deteriorate in a way that has been so damaging to both of us, yet, oddly, I feel like we became a stronger entity as we merged together to try to live with this illness. The verbal wars and daily challenges were really not important to either of us because it was the loftier and unspoken goal of survival that was really taking our attention, and we both knew it.

I have done my best. That's all I can say. We have both done our best.

That is really all I can say.

Year Seven

I swore I wouldn't do this. It was supposed to end back then. It appears that I still need the catharsis of writing. It's January and another new year.

I am despondent, to be sure, and sick. I've been repeatedly sick, it seems. Right now it's a bout of bronchitis with congestion so deep that I rattle whenever I breathe. So, I have camped out in my house for the last four days with the animals at my side to try to recoup some energy. I am too sick to see David this week, so of course that makes it all the worse.

Sometimes now, I just sit in the quiet. I get up in the morning and just sit on the side of the bed for about 15 minutes. Or by some trigger, I will walk to a chair in my living room and just sit. I know this is all about recovery, but I had no idea there would be so much to it, and I had no idea what a painful journey this is, to watch your husband waste away and know that there is nothing you can do. I also had no idea it would be so quiet now.

There has been some peace. I have moved away from the house that David and I shared. I congratulate myself that I had the guts to do it right away and the luck to make it happen. It was a very good decision. I just cannot be consumed with pictures in my mind of David in every room, in every corner of the yard, walking out the door. The day he left on the Council on Aging van for the first time. The day he left his house for the last time. Even now, it hurts to think about these life-changing moments. So, I am in my own place with the dog and two cats and lots of sunshine streaming in the windows. There are trails nearby to walk. I find walking very therapeutic.

✦ ✦ ✦ ✦ ✦ ✦

I have come to know every exit along Route 3 on the long ride up to Chelsea where I go twice a week now. That's where David is. At the Chelsea Soldiers' Home in Chelsea, Massachusetts. The nurse was true to her word and did find David a bed. It took about two more months and came after David had been hospitalized with recurrent intestinal problems and then sent temporarily to a local nursing home. We were at the end of a limited three-week approval for care from our insurance company when I got the call from Chelsea.

I was at the epicenter of having to make a decision about David's care. Only two days before, I had returned to my attorney to start the process for real of applying for Medicaid. Only the previous night, I had stayed up until 3:00 in the morning searching for tax and financial records that I would need for the Medicaid application. The task at hand was nothing but cold reality totally devoid of emotion. I felt like I had been preparing for this moment for years and, suddenly, there it was. David needed care, and we had to ante up anything and everything it would take to provide good care for him.

I will always think of that nurse from Chelsea as an angel descended from heaven to help us when we needed it the most.

It takes six to seven hours for each trip to Chelsea, allowing two hours up, two to three hours with David, and two hours back. In the six, now seven, months he has been there, he has declined so much. He had a major grand mal seizure in June that left him with little language ability and compromised motor skills. I could tell when I got the call saying that he had just been taken by ambulance to the hospital that this was serious business. He was critically ill, and they weren't sure he would survive.

But he recovered and was returned to Chelsea. I am ever so thankful. They are good to him there, sweet to him. He is touched, talked to, smiled at, fed and regularly changed. There has been an extraordinary bonus in long-term care that I did not know would happen—I am now David's partner again, not his caregiver. While I help to feed him when I visit, that's the extent of my care. Anything he needs, the nursing staff is right there to help. They are both proprietary and prideful. His happiness and his physical well-being are in their hands. They are proud of the good work that they do and they should be. They do a great job.

I greet David with a smile and a kiss. His face lights up when he sees me. He will say something that I cannot understand, but we connect with such a depth of love that it restores my faith in God's love and the good things in life. I had so forgotten that life can be good. There are no more frustrations on my part, no more stress and anguish. I am no longer someone who is burdened by caregiving, and that is a gift to both of us.

✦ ✦ ✦ ✦ ✦ ✦

And so here we are. End Stage, as they say. We are now at the difficult crossroads of end-of-life care. His life is now reduced to a geri chair and hospital bed. He no longer walks. He won't eat much solid food anymore. Talking is mostly a mumbo jumbo of words and singsong sounds like an individualized rap. He knows me still. But not my name.

He recognizes me sometimes right away and sometimes not for quite a while, while I sit and hold his hand, rub his back, kiss him, stroke his arm. When he knows me, somehow he manages to tumble out enough words to tell me I am "sooo…byoootiful." Some of the moments he exchanges with his daughters are so poignant, and picture-perfect as well. He grabs onto both of their hands with both of his hands and smiles broadly and tells them as well, "You are sooo…byoootiful."

He also manages to say "I love you" with the emphasis on *love.* The words are mouthed purposefully and slowly. Sometimes it does not sound like "I love you," but I can see as his mouth moves, that that is what he is saying, and he is working hard to say it.

I remember David's mother told me that the name David means *beloved.* I think it was a good name for him. He can still feel the love and that's reassuring. Despite all the things that we cannot control, at least we are all doing enough of the right things for him that he can still feel the love, as we do.

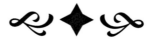

And now it's barely six weeks later. David passed away in mid-February, only nine months after entering the Chelsea Soldiers' Home. We thought he was pretty stable, despite the eating problems. But continuing difficulty swallowing and not eating turned into not drinking. He aspirated sometimes when he tried to drink, and he became dehydrated. Then there was a urinary tract infection and pneumonia. We could have put him on IVs and turned him around, but it would have happened again and again. He would continue to aspirate and it would wreak havoc on his lungs. We chose to allow him a quicker journey, with only a minimum of medications.

The girls and I spent the last seven days with him, by his bedside. Our nephew came to see him for a last visit. We rubbed his back, kissed him, held his hands, helped adjust him in the bed, put tiny sips of water in his mouth. Over several days, I told David the story of our lives together, all the places we had lived and all the wonderful things we had seen and done together. His eyes were half open. He was listening to me. I told him that we were all on vacation, so we had lots of time to spend with him. We were right there with him and we were not leaving.

David was sent to the hospital for a few days with a spiking fever, but I asked to have him moved back to the Chelsea Soldiers' Home. When he was lifted from the ambulance gurney back to his familiar bed at the Soldiers' Home, he opened his eyes wide, and again, and for the last time, mouthed the words *"I love you,"* with the emphasis on *love*. That's the last thing he said to me.

We held on to him when he took his last breath. He did not appear to be in any distress. His breathing simply slowed down and then it stopped and the world became ever so silent.

But things didn't return to normal.

For me, the world will never be normal again. I know that we all live with twists and turns, but for us, it seemed that fate grabbed on to us and refused to let go. In the end, I did not survive normal and neither did David. Our lives were anything but normal.

In the end, all I can say once again is we both did our best. For so long, David laughed his way through his limitations, making up words as he went along, joking and blaming others when things weren't in the right place. For so long, I was mired in anger over being married to someone who had changed so much, who took things so lightly and didn't seem to care about anything beyond the current moment. Then we found out what we were really dealing with. We found out that current moments were all we had, and we would just have to figure out how to live with our reality.

So we did. We figured out how to live with it for as long as we could. Up to the last few days, I could look into David's eyes and feel such a deeply human connection with him. It was beyond love. It was something shared at a cellular level quite apart from our physical selves. When you are dealing with life and death, everything becomes divine, celestial, infinite and passionate. In great defiance of this disease, those feelings survive and will remain with me always.